SalonOvations' Guide to Aromatherapy

SalonOvations' Guide to Aromatherapy

by Shelley M. Hess

Milady Publishing Company
(a division of Delmar Publishers)
3 Columbia Circle, Box 12519
Albany, New York 12212–2519

NOTICE TO THE READER

Cover Design: Brian Yacur
Cover Photo: Stephen Downey

Milady Staff
Publisher: Catherine Frangie
Acquisitions Editor: Marlene McHugh Pratt
Production Manager: Brian Yacur
Project Editor: Annette Downs Danaher
Art/Design Production Coordinator: Suzanne McCarron

COPYRIGHT © 1996
Milady Publishing Company
(a division of Delmar Publishers)

Printed in the United States of America
Printed and distributed simultaneously in Canada

For more information, contact:
SalonOvations
Milady Publishing Company
3 Columbia Circle, Box 12519
Albany, New York 12212-2519

3 4 5 6 7 8 9 10 XXX 05 04 03

Library of Congress Cataloging-in-Publication Data

Hess, Shelley, 1954–
    SalonOvations' guide to aromatherapy / by Shelley Hess.
        p.   cm.
    Includes index.
    ISBN 1-56253-313-4
    1. Aromatherapy—Popular works. 2. Beauty culture—Popular works.
    I. Title.
    RM666.A68H47 1996
    646.7'2—dc20   95-11525
                                                                         CIP

Contents

Acknowledgments

When I was first asked to create this textbook, I decided to investigate all the material that was already published on the subject. The list was long, and filled with great work. Through the guidance of Marlene Pratt, I decided to put all of my successful recipes and treatments—used for years in my personal practice—into book form.

There are several people who I must thank for all of their hard work, encouragement, and support. First, I'd like to thank Marlene Pratt. If it were not for her continual assistance and support, this book would not have been created. Second in line for my gratitude is Annette Danaher, who helped me stay focused on the correct format to make this book a reality.

Third is my sister Jackie. Every writer should be so blessed as to have the genius and creative thought processes that come so naturally to Jackie. Thanks, sis.

Next is Ted Hampton, who allowed me endless amounts of jam-sessions while I worked on my computer through the wee hours of the morning. I appreciate his assistance, love, and support.

Last, but certainly not least, is the entire staff of Milady Publishing Company, for their interest in my work as a holistic health practitioner. None of this would have been possible without their support. Thank you very much.

Thank you also to the following professionals for their expertise and very helpful input while reviewing this manuscript:

Stella Niffenegger, Cincinatti, OH
Jane Kane, Kingston, NY
Haleh Palmer, Schenectady, NY
Holly Williams, Des Moines, IA

Preface

This book is intended to be used as a handbook and guide to aromatherapy. It can be used by all cosmetology professionals, especially hairstylists, estheticians, and manicurists. Specific concentration is provided on the exact applications available for all three disciplines. Detailed information is offered to enable the practitioners to feel confident in their ability to use aromatherapy successfully.

Aromatherapy is a very powerful tool, and the reader will be instructed to consider all the known contraindications, before conducting an aromatherapy treatment. To paraphrase a comment shared with me by Mario Montalvo, a leading cosmetic researcher: aromatherapists will have to understand that essential oils will cause **"crisis healing"**[1] during the first treatments. Crisis healing occurs when the skin/body is quick to detoxify from the use of the essential oils, resulting in the skin surface showing various spots where the toxins have reacted and surfaced. Performing a **"toxicity test"**[2] will help an aromatherapist determine the chance for a client to have a "crisis healing" experience.

To perform a toxicity test, first place your thumb between the natural indent between the two clavicle bones on the décolleté of the client. This natural indented spot between the clavicle bone reflects the thymus gland. It is the thymus gland that handles many of the toxins in the face and body. Gently press your thumb, with a pulsing pressure, three times on this spot. Remove the thumb, look for any redness If it is immediate and definitely flushed, this indicates that the toxin level will be high. This is a good toxicity test.

With every formulation/recipe, exact measurements will be offered. Each professional is expected to follow the recipes as written. The material presented in this book is for the professional's use only. It is not intended for distribution within a salon's clientele for home usage.

Aromatherapy, if used correctly, can be an excellent resource for many successful services within a salon menu list. It can expand the current services being offered at any location. There are no limits to the increase in revenue that aromatherapy treatments can offer. Part of the appeal of adding aromatherapy is the personalizing of every client's service. Added benefits are the pleasant fragrances that will fill the air around the individual work stations.

There has been an increased awareness among consumers about aromatherapy. These consumers may be part of the customer base for salons across the country. Experienced professionals and beauty school graduates need to learn how aromatherapy can affect everyone's lives. Aromatherapy can be an important tool to maintaining the "competitive edge" in the beauty industry.

For your convenience, helpful notes and references are numerically cited in text and explained per chapter in Appendix D: Notes and References.

Shelley M. Hess

About the Author

Shelley Marleen Hess has spent more than 23 years perfecting her knowledge in aromatherapy, holistic health, reflexology, and skin care. Based on her impeccable credentials, she is referred to as one of the consummate holistic professionals in America. Her success as an international author and educator has earned her the position of advisor to the Kirov Ballet Troupe of the former USSR. Her list of professional affiliations include The Society of Cosmetic Chemists; C.I.D.E.S.C.O., USA.; and The National Cosmetology Association's Fashion Committee, Esthetic Division.

Ms. Hess's makeup lesson series, "Putting Your BEST Face Forward" is used as a cosmetology textbook in numerous colleges and has been translated and sold in several countries.

Part 1

Introduction to Aromatherapy

Chapter 1

Definitions

With all the various levels of experience and education found within the beauty industry, this section attempts to outline the most frequently used terms throughout the book; terms that may not be clearly understood by all of the readers.

Definitions of Terms

Acid Rain: a reference to the environmental toxins now found in the ozone layer that pollute the air and are brought down in precipitation (rain and snow).

Alcohol: product of the fermentation of vegetable matter containing sugar. Used in the solvent extraction to create some essential oils.

Allergy: any noxious modification of body fluids caused by some foreign substances.

Alopecia: baldness and/or severe hair loss.

Antibiotic: literally "hostile to life," substances that prevent the development of microbes.

Antiseptic: that which destroys and prevents the development of microbes.

Astringent: agent that causes contraction of organic tissue.

Ayurvedism: The oldest form of medicine, still practiced in many third world countries. Its origins are in India.

Chemotherapy: the specific treatment of disease by the administration of chemical compounds.

Comedone: an impaction inside of the pores on the skin, also referred to as a blackhead.

Compress: method of using essential oils directly on the skin or body part.

3

Cortex: the external layer of an organ. Particularly found on the hair shaft.

Couperose: a French term describing the surface capillaries that are dilated. Often the dilation is permanent.

Crisis Healing: a term used to describe the reaction the skin and body can have to initial essential oil treatments. It references the detoxification capabilities of essential oils as they enter the body.

Décolleté Area: the area of skin that lies on the front of the collar bone and extends to both shoulders and up to the base of the neck.

Dermatitis: inflammation of the dermis.

Dermis: the second layer of the skin. Often called the "true skin." All live cellular activity occurs here. Collagen and elastin fibers are created in this layer.

Eczema: a chronic irritation of the skin, causing a reddening of the tissue.

Edema: a medical term to describe swelling of skin tissue.

Effleurage: A French term describing the type of massage movement that uses the flat part of the fingers and palm of the hand to manipulate the skin and muscles. It is the most popular of all massage movements, and offers the highest degree of relaxation.

Epidermis: the top layer of the skin.

Erythema: skin congestion.

Essential oil: a volatile oily substance produced by many plants. This oil may contain vitamins, hormones, antibiotics and/or antiseptics.

Extraction: used in the making of essential oils, it is a method of separating the oil from the plant or herb. Used in a facial, it is the process of removing comedones and milia from the epidermis.

Heat Rash: a dermatological condition of the skin caused by excessive heat. As the body perspires, the toxins come to the surface and irritate the epidermis causing tiny red bumps to form. It often itches.

Hepatitis: inflammation of the liver.

Hypertension: raised blood pressure.

Lipophilic: used to describe a substance that is attached to fat molecules. These substances will usually mix well in oils.

Milia: a closed impaction, an accumulation of sebum and skin cells trapped in a pore, also referred to as a whitehead.

Nanometer: a scientific measuring device that is so sensitive it has the ability to determine molecular weight by a single cell.

Neat: when using an essential oil, it means that the oil is used directly on any body part.

Olfactory sense: part of the body's senses that relates to smell.

Olfactory nerve: the large, connecting nerve that connects passageways from the top of the nose to the brain. It is one of the strongest, most sensitive nerve endings in the body.

Papule: a clogged pore filled with dead skin cells and sebum. Part of Grade Two acne.

Petrissage: A French term describing a massage movement that kneads the muscles under the skin. It is a bit more forceful in technique than it's partner, effleurage.

Psoriasis: a chronic skin disease characterised by reddish patches with profuse silvery scaling.

Pustule: a papule with bacteria included so that a fluid develops around the clog. The fluid is yellowish and often referred to as pus. Part of Grade Two acne.

Radiation: a medical use of X rays to kill cancer cells.

Sebaceous glands: the glands that produce sebum (oil).

Seborrhea: increased secretion of the sebaceous glands.

Shiatsu: a Japanese word that means finger pressure. It is part of the accupressure massage techniques. Popular because of its gentle, nearly painless style of pressure-point therapy.

Subcutaneous layer: the third layer of the skin. Also known as the hypodermis. All the fat cells are in this layer. It is the natural padding of the skin.

Tapotement: a massage movement using all of the finger tips in unison. Also referred to as the "piano movement."

Toxicity testing: The placing of the thumb between the clavicle bones on the décolleté area, to pre-determine the chance for crisis healing on a new client. It tests the thymus gland's reaction level. It will be quick to redden if the toxin level is high.

Vasoconstrictor: that which contracts blood vessels.

Vasodilator: agent that causes an increase in blood flow.

Vegetation: a plant-like growth that grows from the earth's soil.

Chapter 2

History of Aromatherapy

To grasp the impact that aromatherapy can have on the beauty industry, one needs to understand the impact it has had on the world. It is important to understand its beginnings, as well as its current ability to affect our lives today. Aromatherapy can be as complex or as simple as you want it to be. It is a tool that, if used properly, will provide results in treatments that you did not perceive possible in any other style of application.

Aromatherapy's Timetable of Existence

Aromatherapy may be new to a lot of North Americans, but it is anything but new to civilization. If used properly it has incredible power and will bring about positive changes in the body. The oldest form of medicine is called **Ayurvedism.** To better understand its complexity and thoroughness of application, you would have to research back 10,000 years into India's oldest and most sacred known book, the Vedas. For the reader's knowledge in aromatherapy, this is not necessary. However, it would make fascinating reading.

From the Bible comes references of Moses being directed by God to use myrrh, which was comprised of olive oil and calamus, cassia, and cinnamon. Myrrh is very effective as an antiseptic and stimulator of cell growth.

In the fourth century B.C., Hippocrates was an advocate of using aromatherapy in the bath and in massage oils. He is called the "father of medicine" and he also could be classified as a leader in the use of aromatherapy for medicinal purposes.

As far back as 5000 B.C., the people living in Pakistan used aromatherapy in their communal baths. In 1500 B.C. Egyptians used aromatherapy for deodorants, the priests used it for embalming their pharaohs, and it was also used to heal the mind. Aromatherapy was used for physical and mental therapies with immense success. So much so, that Egyptians and Phoenicians found aromatherapy essences a valuable financial trade. Temples built in Babylonia and India had aromatherapy essences put into the mortar material. It was believed that the aromas would be favorable to the gods. It was in honoring of the gods that "essential oils" had their first widely used purpose. Successful use of essential oils covered parts of the world like Egypt, Israel, India, Greece and Rome. Through battles and conquests, the wonders of aromatherapy traveled throughout the African continent and then to Spain. Through Spain it reached all of Europe and finally into the new world, America.[1]

In the early part of the 20th century, essential oils became the basis for all aromatherapy treatments used today. If the latter part of the 19th century and early 20th century are considered our more recent history, the leaders in developing the use of aromatherapy as it is today hail from Europe. A large representation has come from France and England.

Aromatherapy Pioneers

Although the list is very long, a few are considered the major pioneers and should be mentioned.

Rene-Maurice Gattefosse, a French cosmetic chemist. He wrote one of the first books on aromatherapy. Many consider him to be the first to coin the use of the term "aromatherapy." While working in his own laboratory a serious accident occurred, where he burned his own hand. Choosing to use lavender as a compress, his hand healed faster than anyone expected, and without severe scarring. His work with injured soliders during WWI brought him worldwide acclaim. During this time, he was able to prove the power of penetration of essential oils into the skin. He tracked them in the circulatory system to the lymph. With some of his patients, the penetration took less than an hour, and others it took much longer, up to 10 hours.

Dr. Jean Valnet, also a French physician. He was a pioneer in the medical practice of aromatherapy. His use of essential oils for the treatment of his patients provided him respect in the holistic health field. His work also set the standards of the use of essential oils as direct compresses on almost any part of the body.

Madame Maury, was a notable French woman who brought the field of aromatherapy into the cosmetic and beauty world. Her clinics in England offered beauty students the opportunity to have her hands-on training. Some of her students went on to continue the idea and use of training centers.

Robert Tisserand, from England, opened one of the finest educational centers for the study of aromatherapy in the world today.

Henri Viaud, a perfume distiller from France, perfected the techniques used today to extract the oils from the plants and herbs.

One person who stands out as a leading force in bringing aromatherapy into the United States is Marcel Lavabre. He brought to the states, decades of personal research from his homeland: France. While working his fields and gardens, Marcel perfected cultivation processes of the plants that produced the essential oils. He brought to the United States personal aromatherapy recipes that he worked with. Currently, his company produces and distributes the essential oils that American aromatherapists use in their treatment rooms.

It is important to recognize, that throughout the history of aromatherapy, the majority of uses of aromatherapy were medicinal in nature. The compounds were taken internally.

CAUTION

All usage of aromatherapy treatments in this book will be exclusively external, used only on the hair, nails, and skin!

At no time is the reader to interpret the material in this book is for ingestion or internal use! There can be contraindications about using aromatherapy and its powerful actions. The reader will be advised wherever possible of any widely known contraindications. You are instructed to follow common sense and caution whenever using aromatherapy treatments on any client, for any reason.

Aromatherapy Today

Western civilization has seen advanced medical breakthroughs that have replaced the old methods of the eastern cultures. As technologies became the selected choice of treating people, the traditions of using herbs, roots and plants became passé. The medical communities, at large, began to dismiss the 10,000-year-old ways as relics and nonessential forms of health care. Aromatherapy created the earth's first antibiotics and antiviral treatments. Chemicals and drugs began to look less like their ancestors and more like a factory processed work of art. The elements found in all living plants and roots were somehow immersed in foil-wrapped gel packets and tablets.

Ironically, the processing of essential oils found that the perfumeries and cosmetic factories were still interested in using the essential oils for their topical applications. With the new surge to reduce, reuse or recycle, coupled with the interest of getting back to a healthy environment, essential oils began to find their way into a renewed revelation for the "natural" aides in healing.

Most of the recipes found in this book, may seem to be new and different to the readers. The formulations that the author has been using are recipes taught to her over 20 years ago. And her teachers were taught them decades before then. It kind of fits the old cliche "everything old is new again." Because essential oils are the key element of how aromatherapy fits into the servicing of all clients within the beauty industry, it is important to understand how they affect the body. Essential oils are the vehicle with which the professional uses to perform the treatment to their client. It is through the proper usage of the essential oils that the hairstylist, esthetician, and manicurist reap the rewards of their efforts.

Essential Oils: The Backbone of Aromatherapy Treatments

An extract of plants and roots are what makes an essential oil. The essential oil is very concentrated and fragile to deal with in its raw form. Since all plants and roots need oxygen to survive, the essential oil is quick to evaporate into the air.

Essential oils are considered the inner core of all plants and roots; their heart and soul, so to speak. All the vital life force of the plants and roots are found within the molecules of the singular drops of oil. Essential oils contain the hormones of the plants and roots from which they are extracted. It is through the power of the plants' and roots' life force, that the essential oils can assist the human body's natural defenses. This is accomplished by the essential oils ability to limit the growth of micro-organisms.

Some essential oils have been able to destroy micro-organisms, making these essential oils "nature's antibiotics." Essential oils have a direct healing quality to human hair, skin and nails. All three are comprised of keratin fibers, and essential oils are directly absorbed in keratin. In addition, essential oils play a major role in the molecular structure of the plants' and roots' biochemistry and contribute to their ability to express the natural smells of the plants and roots. Essential oils are "nature's perfumes and fragrances."

An individual molecule of a processed essential oil can be so small that it would register 710 on a **nanometer.** A human skin cell can measure 660. In layman's terms, this means that some processed essential oils are smaller than a human cell, making penetration easy.

Lipophilic Traits

Another element to the success of essential oils' penetration of the skin is that they are **lipophilic.** This means that they have an affinity for fat cells. Since fat cells are found in the subcutaneous layer of the skin, the absorption rate of most essential oils is immediate. The initial effect of essential oils on the human body does not occur in direct contact with the skin, hair and nails.

Effect on Olfactory System

The initial effect is in the **olfactory senses** within our nose and brain. It is through this direct link with the **olfactory nerve** that aromatherapy began to become so popular. Our sense of smell has been proven to be one of our most constant and strongest senses. Tests have been conducted where the brain will register a smell and be able to detect it within two seconds, years after first learning it. The olfactory nerve has a direct link with the center of the brain that controls emotions. With the direct passage connection of the olfactory nerve through the nose, essential oils have had direct responses to people's emotions. Many people have experienced a sense of calm and well-being by walking through a garden. It is the smell of the plants that is providing their brains with the stimulus to have such a reaction.

The professional hairdresser, esthetician and manicurist can promote similar reactions by using essential oils properly. The professional can provide the clients an indispensible tool to bringing about a positive change in clients' behavior during the time that they are in the salon. In turn, this improved attitude will follow them throughout their day or night. Making a positive difference in any of our client's lives, nearly guarantees us a long term relationship with that person. Part of the glory of the beauty industry is knowing that we possess the talents and information to do just that.

We build our reputation and careers on how comfortable our clients feel when they come in for services. Using aromatherapy with your existing customer base will help you gain larger references from them to other potential clients.

Aromatherapy's Aura

Aromatherapy offers an immediate, positive impact on the client the moment they experience it. For centuries aromotherapy's aura (a distinctive atmosphere or subtle sensory stimulus) has been documented as part of its success in bringing about the designated desired changes in the patient. The aura is largely driven through the olfactory nerve, so that it will affect anyone who has direct contact with an individual essential oil.

Now all beauty professionals will be able to tap into the same power of the aromatherapy aura when they use the various aromatherapy treatments designed for their specific area of training. Although there are many differences between hair care, skin care, and nail care, aromatherapy auras will be part of each and every treatment.

Therefore, this book will provide each professional department their specific aromatherapy treatments just for their special needs. However, as a team of professionals working in the same location, they will be able to share their knowledge of aromatherapy to better the entire salon clientele. This way, aromatherapy will be one more way for the salon staff to work together as a team.

Aromatherapy Tomorrow

Aromatherapy will not be a fad or short-lived trend. Aromatherapy has been around the world for more than ten centuries. Considering that the United States of America is only a little more than two centuries old, it is young in comparison to the rest of the world. It has just taken this young country longer to catch up to all the rest. Aromatherapy was used extensively by the American Indian although the early settlers dismissed the knowledge. Now Western medical practices are picking up the information and using the ancient herbs in high-tech research.

With the increase in public awareness of aromatherapy, professionals in all three specialties will increase their usage. The level of excellence in hair care, skin care, and nail care will be judged by the amount of aromatherapy treatments being provided. Aromatherapy will be the guideline for consumers to determine their selection of salons to go to. National beauty magazines, like *Vogue, Elle, Mademoiselle,* and *Glamour* all carry articles about the remedies that aromatherapy treatments provide. As the consumers read these articles, it raises their level of interest. In turn, they will then seek out local experts to help them receive the same treatments written about in the magazines. This author receives phone call inquiries every day about aromatherapy. The callers are always pleased to know that they can come into the salon to get firsthand exposure to aromatherapy.

Aromatherapy treatments are just one way to judge the level of training of any esthetician. There is an increase in the number of estheticians who are seeking advanced training. Although aromatherapy will always have a predominance in skin care, facials, and body care programs, its popularity has enjoyed significant growth in all the other areas of beauty.

Chapter 3

Quick Reference Guide to Essential Oils

This reference guide is a very important part of the book for understanding the complexity of the essential oils. For the novice, this section will have to be read several times. Each time you read it, more of the information will be retained in your memory. Do not let the complexity overwhelm you. Learning about essential oils takes time and a lot of practice. The author hopes that the simplicity of the material will help the readers to gain confidence in their ability to create formulas on their own.

Essential Oils: Common and Latin Names

Each essential oil has a common name and a Latin name. The list gives the common name followed by the Latin name. The Latin name is being offered for those advanced beauty (skin care only) professionals who may want to investigate the medical side of aromatherapy. The Latin name is used more often in the medical community. With the increased awareness of estheticians who want to deal with more medical practices, the Latin terms may be helpful.

This is a fairly comprehensive list. The professionals in the beauty industry WILL NEVER use all of them. Aromatherapy treatments are largely based in the medical practices. Essential oils work for the body and the mind. This book only addresses the part of aromatherapy fitting the TOPICAL/EXTERNAL usage of essential oils. The essential oils listed in **BOLD PRINT**, are the ones most often used, in hair care, skin care and nail care treatments. You should not interpret this to mean that the other essential oils cannot be used. They will, however, only take a greater understanding of all of the components of the client's condition, the condition you are trying to treat, and how the oils will affect or react once entered into the skin, hair, or nails. In dealing with the skin, hair, and nails, it is the hair, *NOT* the scalp, that will have the greatest freedom from a negative reaction.

Essential Oil Names

Common	Latin	Common	Latin
ANGELICA	Angelica archangelic	**JASMINE**	Jasminum officinale
ANISEED	Pimpinella anisum	**JUNIPER**	Juniperus communis
BASIL	Ocimum basilicum	LAVANDIN	Lavandula fragrans
BAY	Pimenta racemosa	**LAVENDER**	Lavandula officinalis
BENZOIN	Styrax benzoin	**LEMON**	Citrus limonum
BERGAMOT	Citrus bergamia	**LEMONGRASS**	Cymbopogon citratus
BIRCH	Betula lenta	**LIME**	Citrus aurantifolia
BLACK PEPPER	Piper nigrum	LOVAGE ROOT	Levisticum officinale
BOIS DE ROSE	Aniba rosaeodora	MACE	Myristica fragrans
CAJEPUT	Melaleuca leucadendron	MANDARIN	Citrus nobilis
CAMPHOR	Cinnamomum camphora	**MARJORAM**	Origanum marjorana
CARAWAY SEEDS	Carum carvi	**MELISSA**	Melissa officinalis
CARDAMOM	Elettaria cardamomum	MUGWORT	Artemisia vulgaris
CARROT	Daucus carota	MYRRH	Commiphora myrrha
CEDARWOOD	Cedrus atlantica	MYRTLE	Myrtus communis
CHAMOMILE-BLUE	Ormensis multicolis	**NEROLI** (orange blossom)	Citrus bagaradia
CHAMOMILE GERMAN	Matricaria chamomilla	**NIAOULI**	Melaleuca viridiflora
CHAMOMILE-MIXTA	Anthemis mixta	NUTMEG	Myristica fragrans
CHAMOMILE ROMAN	Anthemis nobilis	**ORANGE**	Citrus aurantium
CINNAMON BARK	Cinnamonum zeylanicum	OREGANO	Origanum vulgare
CINNAMON	Cinnamomum zeylanicum	**PALMAROSA**	Cymbopogon martini
		PARSLEY	Petroselinum sativum
CISTUS	Cistus landaniferus	**PATCHOULI**	Pogostemon patchouli
CITRONELLA	Cymbopogon nardus	PENNYROYAL	Mentha pulegium
CLARY SAGE	Salvia sclarea	PEPPER	Piper nigrum
CLOVE	Eugenia caryophyllata	**PEPPERMINT**	Mentha piperanta
CORIANDER	Coriandrum sativum	**PETITGRAIN**	Citrus aurantium
CUMIN	Cuminum cyminum	PIMIENTO	Pimienta officinalis
CYPRESS	Cupressis sempervirens	PINE	Pinus sylvestris
DILL	Anethum graveolens	RAVENSARA	Ravensara aromatica
ELEMI	Canarium luzonicum	**ROSE BULGAR**	Rosa damascena
EUCALYPTUS	Eucalyptus globulus	**ROSE MAROC**	Rosa damasacena
EUCALYPTUS LEMON	Eucalyptus citriodora	**ROSEMARY**	Rosmarinus officinalis
EUCALYPTUS PEPPERMINT	Eucalyptus dives	**SAGE**	Salvia officinalis
EUCALYPTUS RADIATA	(same—Eucalyptus dives)	**SANDALWOOD**	Santalum album
		SAVORY	Satureia montana
EVERLASTING	Gnaphalium polycephalum	**SPEARMINT**	Mentha spicata
		SPIKE	Lavandula spica
FENNEL	Foeniculum vulgare	SPRUCE	Picea mariana
FIR	Abies balsamea	**TAGETES**	Tagetes patula
FRANKINCENSE	Boswellia thurifera	TANGERINE	Citrus reticulata
GALBANUM	Ferula galbaniflua	TARRAGON	Artemisia dracunculus
GERANIUM	Pelargonium graveolens	**TEA TREE**	Melaleuca alternifolia
GINGER or GINGER ROOT	Zingiber officinale	THEREBENTINE	Pinus maritimus
		LEMON THYME	Thymus hiemalis
GRAPEFRUIT	Citrus paradisi	RED THYME	Vulgaris thymus
HOPS	Humulus lupulus	THYME	Thymus
HYSSOP	Hyssopus officinalis	VALERIAN	Valeriana officinalis
IMMORTELLE (Italian Everlasting)	Helichrysum angustifolium	LEMON VERBENA	Citroidora lippia
		VETIVER	Vetiveria zizanoides
		VIOLET LEAF	Viola odorata
		YARROW	Achillea millefolium
		YLANG-YLANG	Cananga odorata

NOTE

Although essential oils have the name "oil," they are *not oily*. They have very little slippage by themselves, and a *very small* amount of essential oil is used when doing *any kind of treatment*.

Only the **KEY** essential oils, that are known to work within the beauty industry, will be explored here. All the Latin names have already been listed. The common names are used here. In understanding how to work with essential oils, it is important to grasp the concept of "notes" described below. Essential oils are used for making perfumes and it is for the creation of a perfume that the "notes" are the most important. They determine the final fragrance of the blend of oils. When making a formula for the purpose of an aromatherapy treatment, the "note" is not as important as the action that the essential oil is known to have on the body, skin, nails, and hair.

Categorizing Essential Oils

The essential oil's aroma is important in making the experience a pleasant one for the client. It does not matter if the formula will work if the smell of the mixture sends your client running out the door! There are three categories that all the essential oils fall into. These are: Top notes, middle notes, and base notes. Some oils fall into all three, others in two, but every essential oil will always fit into at least one note level. The classification of these three note levels is very subjective. It is based on how long the natural scent actually lasts. The ultimate test is to place a few drops of any essential oil on a clean, unscented cotton ball, place it in a closed room that is at room temperature (69°F–73°F) and leave it for 24 hours, checking it every 6 hours for the intensity of the aroma. Obviously, this is impractical and unlikely to be accomplished by each individual beauty professional.

Essential oil note classifications are listed below.[1] The reader should use these as a guide and let their own noses be the final judge for themselves.

Top Notes

Essential oils in the top note category are all deep penetrating, sharp smelling, stimulating, uplifting, and volatile in nature. The aroma can last up to 24 hours, however the impact is truly in the first moment of contact. This is the strongest group of essential oils. When they are placed on the surface of the skin, the client experiences either a cold sensation or a hot one. These essential oils do not feel warm. As a rule of thumb, use LESS drops of top notes in the formula. Not all top notes need to be handled in this manner, some of the exceptions are: lemon and petitgrain.

Middle Notes

As the name implies, middle notes are the essential oils that make up the bulk of the formula. They round out the sharpness of the top notes. These aromas can last up to three days. In the formulas these act as equalizers, being able to control the intensity of the more active essential oils. These essential oils have fragrances that people really like, and therefore they often make up at least 50% of the formula.

Base Notes

Base notes make the most lasting impression, since their aromas can last as long as one week. In the formula, the depth and intensity of the base notes deepen and enrich the blend. Many of the essential oils that fall into this category have the ability to penetrate the skin far more thoroughly than all the others. Upon initial contact with the nose, the aroma may not be particularly noticeable, but left on the skin results in a very strong smell. Similar to the way a musk perfume takes awhile to unfold when worn, once it mixes with the chemistry of the skin, it can last longer than other perfumes.

List of Essential Oils

BASIL   (top note) An herb belonging to the Labiate (mint) family. **USE WITH CARE.** An area of confusion in aromatherapy often comes in the use of herbs that are regularly used in food recipes. Basil is a fine example. Basil leaves are placed in cooking water for taste. It is a powerful herb that has many fine properties, but must also be used carefully. It is extracted from the whole plant. Originally from Asia, and now found in France, Cyprus, Madagascar, and the United States.

Other essential oils that blend well are: bergamot, fennel **(remember to only use small amounts of fennel)**, geranium, grapefruit, juniper and lavender.

BENZOIN   (base note) A tree belonging to the Styraceae family. Collected as a resin after cutting the bark. If require benzoin in a liquid form, much more of the tree has to be sacrificed. Native to Thailand and Sumatra, also Borneo and Java.

Other essential oils that work well with it are: carrot, cedarwood, neroli, petitgrain, rose, and sandalwood.

BERGAMOT   (top note) This tree belongs to the Rutaceae family. The oil is expressed from the peel of the fruit off of the tree. Newly ripe fruit is picked in winter for the best oil. 100 kilos of fruit produce 1/2 kilo of oil, which ranges in color from yellow to browny green. Italy is the primary area it comes from, but Morocco and Guinea grow it too.

Other essential oils that work well with it are: cypress, jasmine, lavender, neroli, patchouli, and ylang-ylang.

CAMPHOR   (middle note) Derived from the Asian evergreen tree that belongs to the Lauraceae family. It is extracted in solid form and as an oil, from the camphor found trees naturally in Borneo, China, Japan and Sumatra. In California and Sri Lanka they are cultivated. The oil is not easy to extract.

Other essential oils that work well with it are: clary-sage, cypress, eucalyptus, frankincense, and sandalwood.

CARROT   (middle note) A vegetable in the Umbelliferae family from which the essential oil is obtained from its root and seeds. Primarily grown for aromatherapy in England and France.

Other essential oils that work well with it are: chamomile German, cypress, lavender, and lemon.

CEDARWOOD   (base note) This tree belongs to the Pinaceae family found in North America. Earliest use was by Native Americans who used it as a way to preserve their dead. The essential oil is extracted through steam distillation.

Other essential oils that work well with it are: bergamot, cypress, jasmine, juniper, neroli, and rosemary.

CHAMOMILE GERMAN   (middle note) Also referred to as German chamomile. An herb from the Compositae family. Distilled from Matricaria chamomilla, it has more azulene (an anti-inflammatory and soothing agent) than the others. Which explains its rich blue color. Predominantly from Germany and Hungary. England and South America are cultivating it.

Other essential oils that work well with it are: carrot, geranium, lavender, palmarosa, patchouli, rose, and thyme.

CHAMOMILE ROMAN   (middle note) An herb distilled from *Anthemis noblis* family of dried flowers. Found in Bulgaria, England, France, and Hungary.

It works well with the essential oils that work with the other chamomile (German). Its color is lighter and will change to yellow-brown color when exposed to light.

CINNAMON   (top note) A tree that belongs to the Lauraceae family. The essential oil is extracted from the twigs and leaves. Originated in Madagascar, India and Sri Lanka.

Other essential oils that work well with it are: chamomile German, clove, fennel **(be careful when mixing these two very strong oils),** and geranium.

CLARY SAGE   (top note) An herb from the Labiate family. Found most abundantly in Russia; France and Spain also have cultivated it. The essential oil comes from the tops of the flowers of the plant. It is very sensitive to the way it is grown. Be sure to ask the supplier questions as to its origin.

Other essential oils that work well with it are: cedarwood, geranium, jasmine, juniper, and sandalwood.

CLOVE   (top note) An essential oil that comes from the flower beds of the tree of the Myrtaceae family. Zambia is the best known country to have the trees naturally; but Molucca Islands, the Indies and the Phillipines all cultivate them.

Other essential oils that work well with it are: clary sage, juniper, peppermint, sage, and thyme.

CYPRESS   (middle note) The tree belongs to the Cupressaceae family. The essential oil is extracted from the tree's flowers, twigs and leaves. Germany and France are where they grow naturally, and the Mediterranean cultivate them. Often compared to witch hazel, it is a multipurpose oil.

Other essential oils that work well with it are: chamomile German, juniper, lavender, parsley, pine, and sandalwood.

EUCALYPTUS, EUCALYPTUS LEMON, EUCALYPTUS PEPPERMINT, EUCALYPTUS RADIATA   (top notes) All are trees that belong to the Myrtaceae family. Essential oils are rich, being extracted from fresh leaves. The trees are abundant, growing in Australia, China, Brazil, Spain, Tasmania, and the U.S. (California).

Other essential oils that work well with these are: benzoin, lavender, peppermint, petitgrain, and pine.

EVERLASTING   (top note) A flower from the Compositae family. The essential oil is extracted from the flower tops. Grown throughout Europe. Its aroma has a wide appeal.

Other essential oils that work well with it are: basil, clary sage, pine, and rosemary.

FENNEL (sweet)   (middle note) An herb belonging to the Umbelliferae family. Widely grown worldwide: the United States, Asia, Europe, India, and the Mediterranean.

Other essential oils that work well with it are: basil, cinnamon, geranium, lavender, rose, and sandalwood.

FRANKINCENSE   (base note) A tree that belongs to the Burseraceae family. Originated in East Africa, it has the longest history with Christianity and involved in stories relating the birth of Jesus.

Other essential oils that work well with it are: basil, camphor, geranium, lavender, neroli, orange, and pine.

GERANIUM   (middle note) A plant belonging to the Geranaceae family. Originated in Reunion (a French island in the Indian Ocean), it now flourishes in Algeria, China, Egypt, France, Madagascar, Morocco, and Russia.

Other essential oils that work well with it are: clary sage, frankincense, lavender, rosemary **(use VERY sparingly),** and sage.

GRAPEFRUIT   (middle note) A tree belonging to the Rutaceae family. The essential oil is extracted from the rind of the fruit. Cultivated in Israel and the United States. It is a particularly wide-ranging oil.

There are almost too many other essential oils that work well with it to mention. It works well with most oils. Cedarwood, cypress, lavender, lemon, orange, and parsley are just a few examples.

HYSSOP   (middle note) An herb belonging to the Labiate family. The essential oil is extracted from the flower tops and leaves. Used in biblical times for respiratory treatments. It is a very strong herb, which makes an exceptionally potent oil. Cultivated in Brazil, Europe, and Israel.

Other essential oils that work well with it are: benzoin, chamomile Roman, clary sage, lavender, palma-rosa, rosemary **(remember to use it very sparingly),** and sage.

JASMINE   (base note) A bush that belongs to the Oleaceae family. The essential oil is extracted from the flowers of the bush. Only very small amounts of the oil are required. Cultivated in Algeria, China, Egypt, France, and Morocco.

Like grapefruit oil, this works well with most essential oils.

JUNIPER   (middle note) This bush belongs to the Cupressaceae family. The essential oils are extracted from the dried berries of the bush. The oil is basically colorless, and darkens and thickens as it gets older and exposed to air. Originating in Europe, it now is cultivated in Canada, parts of Africa, and Asia.

Other essential oils that work well with it are: benzoin, clary sage, clove, cypress, lavender, and sandalwood.

LAVENDER   (middle note) This plant belongs to the Labiate family. The essential oil is extracted from the flower tops of the plant. Often mixed with a close member of the same family— Lavandin—to make the oil. The lavandin yields a greater volume than that of the pure lavender. In the lavender plant, the flowers are very fragile, with their tiny star-like shape. Instead of seedlings, cuttings are replanted to cultivate the plant. Originally found in its best form in Provence. Other mountainous areas in England, and Tasmania cultivate the plants.

Other essential oils that work well with it are: carrot, chamomile German, clary sage, patchouli, pine, rose, and rosemary **(remember to use sparingly, and NEVER during pregnancy).**

LEMON   (top note) This tree belongs to the Rutaceae family. The essential oil is extracted from the rind of the fruit. Originally hand-cared for in Sicily, this essential oil made Italy the center of all the lemon oil industry. Though prepared by machines, hand processing still makes the richest essential oil. By 1887, it was brought over from Europe to the U.S. (California) and later to Florida.

Lavender and neroli are just two of the many other essential oils that work well with lemon.

LEMONGRASS   (top note) This grass belongs to the Poaceae family. The essential oil is extracted from the whole wild grass. Cultivated in some parts of Africa, Brazil, Madras, Sri Lanka and West Indies. It is harvested from midsummer to midwinter. It takes a great deal of lemongrass to extract the essential oil (approximately 100 kilos to extract approximately 20 kilograms). With the color similar to what dry sherry looks like, its natural aroma is very strong and resembles a lemon.

Other essential oils that work well with it are: basil, cedarwood, geranium, jasmine, lavender, orange, and oregano.

LIME   (top note) This tree belongs to the Rutaceae family. The essential oil is extracted from the rind of the fruit. Brazil, Italy, Mexico and West Indies cultivate the tree. California and Florida began cultivation of lime in the late nineteenth century.

Other essential oils that work well with it are: bergamot, jasmine, mandarin and orange.

MARJORAM   (middle note) This herb belongs to the Labiate family. The essential oil is extracted from the flower tops and leaves. Originating from Egypt, it is now widely cultivated in Spain, France, Germany, Hungary, and Portugal. If you purchase the essential oil from Spain, make sure to use its Latin name (origanum majorana), because the Spanish refer to their Spanish thyme (*thymus mastichina*) as "marjoram" and although it, too, is an essential oil, it is not the same oil, nor is it used for the same reasons.

Other essential oils that work well with it are: benzoin, bergamot, cypress, lavender, petitgrain, and rosemary **(remember to use sparingly whenever selecting rosemary for any reason or blend).**

MELISSA   (middle note) This herb belongs to the Labiate family. More commonly referred to as balm oil. It originated in Europe and is cultivated in the Mediterranean. The essential oil is extracted from the leaves of the herb, but yields such small quantities of oil that its use is limited due to its extremely high price and limited supply. It has a strong positive effect on people. It is the first choice to make people feel happier, though usually in a highly adulterated form (with other oils) since it is so expensive.

Other essential oils that work well with it are: geranium, lavender, neroli, and ylang-ylang.

MYRRH   (base note) This tree belongs to the Burseraceae family. The essential oil is extracted as a gum resin from the bark of the tree. All essential oils are all considered to be the hormone of the plant, herb, or tree, however this essential oil is a hormonal oil. This essential oil is especially recognized from its relationship with biblical history.

Other essential oils that work well with it are: basil, camphor, cypress, eucalyptus, lavender, niaouli, and thyme.

NEROLI   (top note) The tree belongs to the Rutaceae family. The exact tree is the bitter orange tree. It is a close relation to the sweet orange tree, which makes a different essential oil. This essential oil is extracted from the flower petals. Originating in Italy, where it got its name, it is cultivated in Egypt, France, Morocco, and Tunisia. The oil obtained from France is of extreme high quality.

Other essential oils that work well with it are: benzoin, bergamot, clary sage, geranium, jasmine, lavender, and orange.

NIAOULI   (top note) This bush belongs to the Myrtaceae family. The essential oil is extracted from the leaves and twigs of the bush. It is cultivated in Australia, East Indies, and Tasmania.

Other essential oils that work well with it are: clary sage, eucalyptus, geranium, lavender, myrrh, patchouli, and tea tree.

ORANGE   (top note) This tree belongs to the Rutaceae family. The essential oil is extracted from the rind of the fruit. Two other essential oils (neroli and petitgrain) are obtained from this tree, but extracted from different parts. Originating in China, it is now cultivated in Brazil, France, Spain and the United States (California and Florida). Always make sure that the orange essential oil that you use is of top quality. A key test for this is its natural orange color.

Other essential oils that work well with it are: cedarwood, geranium, ginger, lemon, lime, neroli, and petitgrain.

OREGANO   (middle note) This herb belongs to the Labiate family. The essential oil is extracted from the flower tops and leaves. Cultivated in Africa, Asia, Egypt, and Europe.

Other essential oils that work well with it are: grapefruit, juniper, lemongrass, and parsley.

PALMAROSA   (middle note) This grass plant belongs to the Graminae family. The essential oil is extracted from the whole plant. Cultivated in Brazil and Central America.

Other essential oils that work well with it are: carrot, chamomile Roman, hyssop, patchouli, and sandalwood.

PARSLEY   (base note) An herb that belongs to the Labiate family. The essential oil is extracted from the seeds of the plant. Cultivated throughout Europe.

Other essential oils that work well with it are: cypress, geranium, grapefruit, and sage.

PATCHOULI   (base note) A plant belonging to the Labiate family. The essential oil is extracted from the young leaves. As the plant matures, it loses the ability to make the oil. Originated in the Philippines. It is cultivated in China, Indonesia, Madagascar, and Japan.

Other essential oils that work well with it are: bergamot, geranium, lavender, myrrh, and neroli.

PEPPERMINT   (top note) This herb belongs to the Labiate family. The essential oil is extracted from the whole plant. The flower tops create the better oil. Cultivated in China, England, throughout Europe, and in the United States. England has the reputation of providing the finest peppermint oils.

Other essential oils that work well with it are: benzoin, cedarwood, lemon, myrrh, rosemary **(remember to use sparingly and NEVER during pregnancy),** and tea tree.

PETITGRAIN   (top note) This tree belongs to the Rutaceae family. This is the bitter orange tree that produces neroli from its flowers, and this essential oil is extracted from the leaves and twigs. Therefore Petitgrain is not as potent as neroli, its sister oil. Cultivated in Africa, Brazil, France, Italy and Paraguay. The French have the reputation of producing the finest petitgrain oils.

Other essential oils that work well with it are: carrot, chamomile Roman, geranium, lavender, lemon and palmarosa.

ROSE BULGAR and **ROSE MAROC**   (base notes) These rose bushes belong to the Rosaceae family and are grown in two different countries: Bulgaria and Morocco. Their essential oils are extracted from the flower petals. It takes so many petals to create the oil that the pure oil is very expensive. Due to the large amounts of flowers it takes to make just one drop of pure oil, rose water is used more often. The potent aroma of rose oil makes it one of the most powerful and loved.

The list of other essential oils that work well with these can be almost endless, for these two oils are extremely flexible for blending, a partial list would look like this: bergamot, chamomile, clary sage, cypress, geranium, jasmine, juniper, parsley, patchouli, and sandalwood.

ROSEMARY   (middle note) This herb belongs to the Labiate family. The essential oil is extracted from the flower tops from the plant and the leaves. The flower tops create a purer oil. It originated in Spain. It is cultivated in France, Japan, Tunisia, and what used to be called Yugoslavia. Tunisia has the reputation of producing the finer oil. Rosemary is extremely powerful and can be highly toxic. Part of what contributes to its volatile nature is that sage, spike and turpentine can be used to adulterate the composition of the oil, thus reducing its purity.

Other essential oils that work well with it are: basil, cedarwood, frankincense, lavender, and peppermint.

SAGE   (top note) This herb belongs to the Labiate family. The essential oil is extracted from the sun-dried leaves and flower tops from the plant. The purer oil comes from the flower tops. Originating in the Mediterranean, it is cultivated in China. Its natural yellow color tends to make one believe it will smell sweet, when in reality the aroma mimics camphor.

Other essential oils that work well with it are: lemongrass, sandalwood, and violet leaf oil.

SANDALWOOD   (base note) This tree belongs to the Santalaceae family. The essential oil is extracted from the heart of the center of the tree. This means that the oil is only available when the tree is old and ready to be cut down. This has a direct impact on the price of the oil, due to its limited availability. It can take more than three decades for a tree to mature. The trees grow in India and Indonesia.

Other essential oils that work well with it are: benzoin, cypress, frankincense, juniper, neroli, palmarosa, rose bulgar, rose maroc, and ylang-ylang.

SPEARMINT   (top note) This herb belongs to the Labiate family. The essential oil is extracted from the plant's flower tops and leaves. The flower tops produce the purer oil. It is cultivated in Europe, the Mediterranean, Soviet Union and the United States.

Other essential oils that work well with it are: basil, lavender, parsley, and petitgrain.

TAGETES   (base note) This essential oil is extracted from the plant's flowers. Cultivated in France and Africa. Also referred to as marigold, it has a brownish-orange color.

Other essential oils that work well with it are: eucalyptus-lemon, lavender, lemon, myrrh, and tea tree.

TEA TREE   (top note) This tree belongs to the Myrtaceae family. The essential oil is extracted from the leaves and twigs of the tree. Cultivated in Australia, China, India, and Tasmania. Australia has the reputation of producing the best oil. Although the name tea tree is misleading, it is not a tea, as we know tea to be.

Other essential oils that work well with it are: chamomile German, cypress, lemon, myrrh, neroli, and orange.

THYME (Sweet and Lemon)   (top notes) These are herbs and belong to the Labiate family. The essential oils are extracted from the flower tops and leaves from the plant. The flower tops produce the better quality oil. Cultivated in the Mediterranean.

NOTE

It is important to know the exact kind of thyme you are purchasing. They are not all the same.

In fact, **red thyme** must be avoided for all young children, and for many adults, due to its powerful composition of phenol. All thyme has some alcohols and phenols, but the sweet and lemon variations can be successfully incorporated into beauty care products.

Other essential oils that work well with it are: bergamot, cedarwood, grapefruit, lemon, melissa, rosemary **(remember to use with care, and NEVER during pregnancy),** and sage.

VIOLET LEAVES   (middle note) This plant belongs to the Labiate family. The essential oil is extracted from the leaves of the plant. Cultivated in England, France, Greece and Italy. England is known for the quality of its oil.

Other essential oils that work well with it are: benzoin, carrot, cypress, fennel **(remember that only a very small amount is used),** neroli, and rose bulgar/rose maroc.

YLANG-YLANG   (base note) This tree belongs to the Annonaceae family. The essential oil is extracted from the blooming flowers of the trees. Early summer is when the flowers are best to harvest, although they are gathered year-round. There are several grades of oil, and the best and lightest molecular portions are taken away for expensive and exotic perfumes. The rest are then available for aromatherapy purposes. Unfortunately, these grades do not have as pleasant an aroma. Therefore, in aromatherapy, this essential oil does not have as wonderful an experience as the perfumes. Cultivated in the Comoro Islands, Indonesia, and the Philippines. Manila has the reputation of creating the best ylang-ylang oils.

Other essential oils that work well with it are: bergamot, clary sage, frankincense, jasmine, lavender, lemon, neroli, orange, and sandalwood.

Carrier/Base Oils

Not to be confused with the "base note," a base oil or carrier oil is the substance used to "carry" the essential oil into the body. The terms "base oil" and "carrier oil" are used interchangeably.

As mentioned before, some essential oils possess the full range of notes. Jasmine and ylang-ylang are just two examples of essential oils that have all three characteristics. These two, along with the others, such as rose, can be used alone with a carrier oil. All essential oils are mixed with one carrier/base oil.

The base oil works as the vehicle for essential oils to be massaged into the specific body part, hair, scalp, skin, and nails. There are 17 different carrier/base oils:

1. almond oil	10. jojoba oil
2. apricot kernel oil	11. olive oil
3. avocado oil	12. peanut oil
4. borage seed oil	13. safflower oil
5. hazelnut oil	14. sesame oil
6. carrot oil	15. soya bean oil
7. corn oil	16. sunflower oil
8. evening primrose oil	17. wheatgerm oil
9. grapeseed oil	

Part of why aromatherapy can be so complicated, is that each carrier oil has its own reaction to the skin, hair, and nails. Some, such as avocado or hazelnut, will penetrate more quickly. Some, like wheatgerm, will be more nourishing to the skin. Do not get overwhelmed. Many of the oils, such as almond, corn, grapeseed, olive, peanut, soya bean and sunflower, react very much in the same manner. Their differences are in their specific aromas.

As you become more comfortable with aromatherapy treatments, you will find some of the carrier oils easier to work with than others. Some will have a more pleasant "feel" to them, along with having their own aroma. Not everyone will get the same reaction to the various carrier oils. Experimentation is the best way to find what suits you and your clients.

Besides selecting the carrier oil based on "feel," and "smell," the third and possibly the most controlling factor will be "price." Not all the carrier oils are the same. When letting price be the deciding factor, make sure the base oil is 100% pure.

When creating an aromatherapy formula, try to make up what will be needed for the day. The vegetable base oils keep fairly well alone; however, once the essential oils are added, the mixture will turn rancid as it oxidizes. To keep the solution from turning bad, add enough wheatgerm oil into the mixture to make up only 5% of the complete formula.

In Appendix A at the end of the book is a list of suppliers of aromatherapy oils and equipment. Do not hesitate to ask them as many questions about the processing of the products as necessary to insure your confidence in the quality of the materials. Creating the essential oils is a long and complicated process. A partial description of available stock/parameters is provided in the supplier's section.

Primary Uses of Essential Oils

Some general misconceptions can easily be created in the minds of the newcomers to aromatherapy. Most of the essential oils are derived from natural food sources. It would be easy to mistake the potency of the essential oil, if the potency is based on how often we would find the plant, fruit, or vegetable on our dinner plate. Using any essential oil is using the strongest, most volatile part of the plant, fruit, or vegetable. The concentrations are unequal and can NOT be paralleled to the amount served in a recipe for a meal. The Golden Rule for using essential oils is: LESS WILL ALWAYS BE THE BETTER CHOICE.

BASIL   (**CAUTION:** Use with care.) Although this herb is used in many food recipes, do NOT misinterpret it to be a gentle aromatherapy oil.

Primary use: To unclog congested, sluggish skin. Works as a natural insect repellent.

BENZOIN   "Friar Balsam" is a common nickname for this essential oil.

Primary use: To regenerate mature, inelastic skin. It helps to moisturize dry skin. Also good for chapped, dry and cracked hands. As in all base notes, it is warm and sedating to the skin. The clients should enjoy this essential oil as it is being massaged on them.

BERGAMOT   (**CAUTION:** Extra care must be used, because the oil makes the skin photosensitive.) Bergamot is never to be used directly on the skin. It is strongly suggested that the clients wear sunscreens on areas bergamot is to be used. Apply sunscreen before applying bergamot.

Primary use: For all oily skin and hair, and seborrhea of the scalp. Acne conditions and rosacea also respond well to it. IF you know that the client is an active outdoors person and will NOT use sun protection, choose another essential oil for your formula. The practitioner who uses this essential oil as part of their treatment, must also protect their own hands with a sunscreen.

CAMPHOR   (**CAUTION**: It must not be used during pregnancy.) Very small amounts should be used. The Golden Rule particularly applies to this essential oil. Where 4–5 drops of other oils would be fine, 1–3 drops will do nicely for this one.

Primary use: For oily skin and hair. If used, is generally included in products that are washed off; such as cleansers, shampoos, and masks rather than moisturizers.

CARROT   This essential oil has the power to stain the skin, nails, and scalp. Care must be taken not to use it "neat" (straight on the skin).

Primary use: For all skin, hair, and nail care that needs revitalizing and moisturizing. It also has a calming effect on the skin and cuticles.

CEDARWOOD   With its natural woodsy aroma, this essential oil will appeal to men and anyone else who enjoys the smell of the outdoors. However, clients who have allergies to wood spurs and other forest elements, will not do well with this essential oil.

Primary use: Hair care: this essential oil is helpful in treating alopecia, dandruff, and seborrhea of the scalp. Skin care: for oily skin and irritations.

CHAMOMILE GERMAN   It is particularly mild and gentle and can be used on young children. The practitioner will find that this essential oil has broad appeal for its natural aroma and versatile usage.

Primary use: For all skin and nails that are sensitive, dry, or irritated. With nails, if they are cracked and chapped, this essential oil is very effective. Use on scalps that are dry or flaky. Capillary distention such as couperose, is helped. It will also soothe acne and eczema.

CHAMOMILE ROMAN   Used similarly to chamomile German, above. It also shares its treatment selection variety and broad appeal.

CINNAMON   A very potent essential oil. USE VERY SPARINGLY. Too much in skin potions can cause irritations. Not to be used "neat," or unadulterated. It performs well in blends where it is just a small part of the formula.

Primary use: Skin and nail care. It works very well to tone the skin, and as an antiviral in skin and nails.

CLARY SAGE   This herb is a winner with all aromatherapists. It works very quickly on the body, in many different applications. It does not have a strong positive or negative response to its aroma. It is not a scent that is widely recognized upon first contact.

Primary use: On mature skin to perk up the complexion, as a cell regenerator. It soothes any skin or nails that are inflamed. Stimulates hair growth and helps to regulate seborrhea of the scalp.

CLOVE   A very powerful and potent essential oil, so USE ONLY THE TINIEST OF DROPS. Most people are aware of it as a spice in cooking. And many will have a predetermined idea as to whether they like its natural aroma. Check with your client first, before deciding to select this as part of a blended formula.

Primary use: Helps fight bacteria in nails and skin.

CYPRESS   Another woodsy aroma that will have a certain appeal to "outdoor lovers." But check with your client on the possibility of their having allergies to tree pollens, before selecting this oil.

Primary use: Toning the body, balancing oily skin, strengthening nails. Works as an antiseptic to all skin and nails, oxygenates broken capillaries.

EUCALYPTUS, EUCALYPTUS LEMON, EUCALYPTUS PEPPERMINT, EUCALYPTUS RADIATA (**CAUTION:** Do not use on young children, or anyone with even the mildest asthmatic condition.) This oil's aroma does not blend in with other essential oils' aromas. It will always dominate the blend's smell. One drop of this essential oil can equal the aroma power of 10 drops of other less aromatic selections. Once again, check with your client's preference to its smell. Many will relate its aroma to medicinal products used in their youths.

Primary use: Acne and oily skin. Great for increasing the circulation of the nail beds and cuticles. Superb scalp stimulator. An excellent antiseptic.

EVERLASTING Similar to eucalyptus, this oil's aroma does not blend in with the aromas of other essential oils. It will always dominate the blend's smell. Once again, check with your client's preference to its smell.

Primary use: It has strong anti-inflammatory properties that are wonderful on sensitive skin, acne conditions, or any inflamed nails, cuticles, or skin. If the scalp gets inflamed after a chemical service, it will aide in reducing the redness.

FENNEL (sweet) (**CAUTION:** Use with care, and never during pregnancy.) Inside of the herb is a high phenolic ether content, thus a VERY VERY small amount is to be used in the formula. It is hard to predict your client's response to the aroma. It will go either way. Most often, the formula will only have one drop of this essential oil. The Golden Rule ALWAYS fits this oil.

Primary use: For cleansers for oily skin. To revitalize mature skin and hands.

FRANKINCENSE Not as pungent as eucalyptus, still it will dominate the blends's aroma. Check your client's preference. It will not be as recognizable as eucalyptus. Only the more advanced practitioners will find themselves turning to this essential oil a lot.

Primary use: Skin: For calming any inflamed tissue and for toning loose skin. Nails: Excellent for treating damaged cuticles. Hair: Adds body to limp hair.

GERANIUM   Its natural aroma has broad appeal to women of all ages. Most often men will find the aroma of this essential oil "too flowery." They might think that you are covering them in a woman's perfume.

Primary use: Multifunctional. Can be effective as a cell generator for mature skin, an astringent for oily skin, and decrease the slick found on acne skin. Offers quick repair for chapped, cracked hands and cuticles. Helps reduce the "greasy" hair sensation.

GRAPEFRUIT   It has large universal appeal, partly due to its overwhelmingly popular aroma, and for its wide-ranging abilities.

Primary use: Uniformly used for hair, skin, and nails. No one area is stronger than the others. Hair: It reduces the slick formed by seborrhea and reduces dandruff scales. It increases the fresh bounce to most hair. Skin: It works with toning facial and body tissue, especially tissue with cellulite. Nails: It brightens yellow nails, helps increase the oxygen flow to nails to rid buildup of residue on the nail beds. It strengthens the cuticle tissue.

HYSSOP   (**CAUTION:** Must be used with care, because it is so strong an oil. It cannot be used during pregnancy.) This herb's natural aroma may not be on everyone's top ten list. Check with your client first. Very small amounts of oil are used in any formula. For most formulas, the maximum amount of drops will be two.

Primary use: For moisturizing any sensitive skin and reducing redness of couperose. Excellent for treating eczema of the scalp and skin. Will treat hands and feet for weak nails or damaged cuticles.

JASMINE   A solvent must be used to extract the oil out of the flower. Often ether is the chosen solvent. The process creates an increase in the financial pricing of the end product, the essential oil. Careful selection of the pure absolute of the jasmine flower will assure the proper oil for use. Only very small amounts of the oil are required. This flower has a strong oriental aroma, and the reaction to it will be close to 50–50 positive or negative. Clients who suffer greatly from hayfever-style allergies might not have a positive reaction to this oil.

Primary use: It has exceptional versatility. In some formulations it will reduce the oily slick off of skin and hair. While in other formulations it can be an overall moisturizer for dry skin, scalp, and nails. Due to its gentle nature, it works well with all sensitive bodies, hands and feet.

JUNIPER   In ancient times it was the antiseptic of choice. It was considered the "rubbing alcohol" of the aromatherapy world.

Primary use: Still used as an active antiseptic for all skin and body areas, including the hands and feet. It is often part of the toning formulations for treating cellulite and flabby arms. In skin care, many acne conditions are improved and oily skin reduces its sebum levels.

LAVENDER   Its aroma makes this essential oil very popular with all ages. It has a fine calming reaction to the internal and external parts of the body.

Primary use: This essential oil can be used on all parts of the body, even the eyes and lips. Hair: To treat alopecia and dry, brittle hair. Skin: Acne, rosacea and oily skins respond well to lavender. Most inflammation of the skin, as well as psoriasis, is reduced. On mature skin, it aids in moisture. For the hands and feet: it works beautifully to soothe and relieve chapping and cracking.

LEMON: (**CAUTION:** Keep away from area directly around the eyes.) It tops the list of the most favored essential oil, due to the powerful aroma of the fruit and its wide appeal with men and women alike. It would be very hard to find a person that does not like the natural fragrance of this oil.

Primary use: One of the most flexible oils of all. It can be used on every body part from the top of the scalp and hair, to the bottoms of the feet. Depending on how it is mixed, it works with oily or dry skin. It energizes the mature skin and repairs wrinkled skin to a new smoothness. For nails it clears yellowing and refreshes the nail beds and cuticles. Whether you are a beginning or an advanced practitioner, you will find that you use this essential oil often.

LEMONGRASS: (**CAUTIONS:** Do not use this on children. Do not use directly on the skin. Do not use on clients allergic to grass or pollens.) This essential oil is known for its antiseptic properties. However, it does have the ability to act as an irritant if applied directly on the skin. It should NOT be used DIRECTLY on the skin—straight, also known as "neat." In blends, use just a little bit of this essential oil. For most formulas, do not go over the four drop level.

Primary use: Predominantly used in body care, for toning, and as an antiseptic. Also used on oily or acne skin to reduce pustules—BUT only as a blend, not straight on its own.

LIME   (**CAUTION:** Keep away from the eyes.) A close choice to its "cousin" the lemon, its natural aroma is strongly popular with men. It is not as diversified as the lemon and not used as often.

Primary use: On the skin as an astringent and tonic.

MARJORAM   Although it is colorless, it is also very pungent. It does not appeal to everyone. Check with your clients before selecting this essential oil for your blend.

Primary use: For treating bruising of any tissue or black-and-blue marks on the scalp, skin, hands, and feet. For damaged nail beds, such as "blackened nails," it has a positive healing quality.

MELISSA   Clients will either find this essential oil very pleasant smelling or be repelled by its aroma. Check with the client first before making your blend.

Primary use: Nails and feet: It is a wonderful antifungal solution. Skin: Depending on the blend of the formula, acne and eczema are aided, and mature skin can be regenerated. This essential oil can be custom fit into oily or dry skin treatments.

MYRRH   A hormonal oil, this essential oil is highly recognized for its involvement in biblical history. Due to its connection, this oil has a strong aura surrounding it. Clients may respond from a deep emotional reaction to this oil, solely based on its connection to Jesus.

Primary use: Skin care: Regenerates and revitalizes mature skin. For skin that is red and sore looking, it acts as an anti-inflammatory. Nails: Reduces redness in dry, cracked hands and cuticles. Hair: Acts as an anti-inflammatory oil for scalps.

NEROLI   It has a pale yellow color. Its aroma is particularly strong and will be pleasant to many people.

Primary use: Hair: Treats scalps that are sore, or cracked and picked at. Nails: Treats bitten and torn cuticles or reddened, cracked hands and feet. Skin: Treats skin that is showing signs of irritation. This oil is perfect for treating sensitive skin.

NIAOULI   Its natural aura is very similar to lavender, which makes it very popular with most people.

Primary use: As a broad spectrum antiseptic solution. Skin: Improves acne and oily skin. Feet: Treats any cuts and sores.

ORANGE   It is very mild, which makes it a good choice for children and anyone with sensitive skin. Its aroma makes it one of the most popular essential oils. From the beginners to the advanced, this essential oil will be chosen often.

Primary use: Hair: It makes the hair silky smooth and shiny. Nails: It is perfect for treating rough, dry hands and feet. If the skin is weak and flabby-looking, it will revitalize it. Skin: Reduces the oil on oily and acne conditions. It helps treat congested skin. On mature skin, it improves tone and smoothness.

OREGANO   (**CAUTION:** Must be used sparingly.) This is a strong essential oil. The aroma is so connected to food, that your clients may actually get hungry when the blend is created. It has broad appeal for both men and women.

Primary use: Body: It works very well on cellulite. Nails: It brightens the nail beds.

PALMAROSA   This essential oil is extremely versatile. The only possible limitation will be for clients with allergies to pollens and grasses. The aroma is neither engaging nor repelling.

Primary use: Hair: It is effective in reducing limp hair. Nails: Revitalizes dry, cracked hands and nails. Also for tired feet that are dry and flaky. Skin: It energizes mature, wrinkled skin.

PARSLEY   This essential oil's appeal is based on its overall acceptance in food preparation. It helps the body clear itself of toxins.

Primary use: An effective antiseptic for skin, nails and feet. Skin: It is effective on couperose and it tones skin. Hair: It helps rid cigarette toxins from the follicles.

PATCHOULI   This oil has the ability to perform two different actions based on the quantity of the oil. Very few drops will energize, whereas many drops will relax. The exact reason is not known.

Primary use: As part of its ability to work in different reactions: it is excellent for cracked, dry hands and feet. Skin: Oily and acne skin conditions are improved and put back into balance. Hair: Restores body to oily hair.

PEPPERMINT   A very powerful essential oil, partly due to its cellular composition and partly due to its aroma. A strong favorite with young clientele. It can overwhelm the formula if its percentage of drops is significantly higher than the others. However, it can also create a popular aroma when mixed with other essential oils that have aromas that are not as pleasant.

Primary use: A major aid in reducing inflammation, irritation, and couperose. Ashy coloring of skin from smoking or prolonged sickness will brighten. On oily or acne skin, it helps reduce the congestion. Hair: It is a major tool in stimulating the scalp and loosening scales of dandruff and eczema. Nails: With its ability to oxygenate the area, it helps nails restore a healthy coloring.

PETITGRAIN   It is not as favorable in aroma to its sister oil, neroli.

Primary use: It works as a great balancer for oily conditions. Skin: Reduces oily sebum slicks and waxy buildup on acne skin. Hair: Reduces the greasy sensation on hair and scalp.

ROSE BULGAR and **ROSE MAROC**   The potent aroma of rose oil makes it one of the most powerful and loved by women and not favored by most men. It is so gentle that it can be used on the most sensitive skins and on very young children.

Primary use: For treating all sensitive skin that is dry. On mature skin it helps reduce the signs of aging. On oily skin it reduces redness. It has a calming effect on any couperose. It soothes rough, cracked, and dry conditions on hands and feet.

ROSEMARY   (**CAUTION:** Because it naturally possesses ketones of camphor, never use it under any conditions on a pregnant woman.) This essential oil will frighten the beginner, though it is NOT an oil that the practitioner should stay away from. Rather it is suggested that care and understanding be used. Ask questions of your supplier to assure that the oil is pure. Do not let the "purse strings" determine which oil is purchased. The best rosemary oil will be costly and worth it! It is a natural cleanser of toxins, reducer of sebum, and a cellular regenerator. This makes this essential oil one of the most diverse.

Primary use: Hair: Alopecia, dandruff, and seborrhea of the scalp all improve with use. Skin: Oily plugs and acne conditions lessen. On mature skin the cells perk up, become less wrinkled. Nails: Feet and hands will gain smoothness and increase in circulation with use.

SAGE (**CAUTION:** It should not be used on pregnant women.) Be careful when using sage in a blend. Its aroma may not mix well with everything.

Primary use: Hair: It is effective in reducing alopecia. Skin: It works to unclog congested skin, or improve skin that has a tendency to be sluggish.

SANDALWOOD The woodsy aroma makes it particularly popular with men and many actively outdoor-loving women. It would be wise to check if the client has a history of allergies to grasses, trees and pollens, before choosing this oil.

Primary use: It works as a terrific antiseptic and antifungal solution. Nails: This is great for any nail care needs when dealing with fungus. Skin: Perfect for treating dry, cracked hands or feet. It also works on dry, mature, wrinkled conditions. Hair: It is added to solutions to make brittle hair have more moisture.

SPEARMINT Its minty aroma makes it a hit with most people. It has an uplifting effect to clients just walking in. Some salons choose to use this oil as a natural fragrance to brighten up the atmosphere.

Primary use: Besides using its natural aroma to uplift the room, it is used as a body toning oil.

TAGETES (**CAUTION:** This essential oil, must be used with extreme care. It is toxic if used directly on the skin, hands and feet. Never use during pregnancy, it has a naturally abortive reaction.)

Primary use: With all the warnings of its being toxic, if used in a very diluted blend, it is extremely effective when treating athlete's foot and any fungal infections of the nails.

TEA TREE This essential oil has a very pungent aroma and, by itself, is not particularly appealing. It has strong antiseptic and antifungal properties, and works well in all areas of the body.

Primary use: Hair: On the scalp it is very effective in controlling dandruff and any irritations. Skin: Improves acne conditions and reduces excess sebum. It is one of nature's best ointments for herpes. Nails: It works incredibly well to control nail fungus.

THYME (Sweet and Lemon) Both oils work very well as antibiotics, antiseptics, and antifungals.

Primary use: Due to their special properties, they are extremely effective during a pedicure. Treats any fungal infections on the nails, hands and feet. Used as an antiseptic for the scalp and skin.

VIOLET LEAF   It has a very light and pleasant aroma, which makes it particularly favorable with mature women. It is a relatively mild oil.

Primary use: Skin and nails: It is used to moisturize skin on the body, face, hands, and feet. It softens the appearance of wrinkles on mature skin.

YLANG-YLANG   The grades of oil available for aromatherapy are of a lesser quality. They tend to resemble jasmine in fragrance, although not quite as distinct. Its aroma can be repelling to some; therefore, check with your client before adding it to the blend. As in all tree oils, check for allergies to tree pollens before deciding to use this essential oil.

Primary use: Hair: It helps to degrease oily hair and scalp. Skin: Can help control acne and oily skin conditions. Nails: During pedicures, ylang-ylang acts to soften rough calluses.

Hair and Scalp Care Formulas: General Guidelines

NOTE
When creating any formula, always keep in mind and/or review the previous sections detailing the characteristics of essential oils, "note" categories, and carrier/base oils.

There are three major considerations to take into account when making up the formulations.

1. Is it for the scalp or hair?
2. If for the hair, how long is it?
3. How sensitive is the client's scalp?

The longer the hair, more product will be needed. The more sensitive the scalp, the milder the formulation. Although not always the case, the fewer the drops of essential oil determines the strength of the solution. In the case of essential oils such as rosemary, fennel, and clove, few drops are always used. When working on the scalp, less solution is created than is with the hair. The area is smaller, so less product is needed.

Aromatherapy Shampoo Formulas

Begin with two ounces of the base. In most cases this will be a mild, unscented, pH-balanced shampoo.

When mixing in the essential oils, always keep the blend to no more than four different essential oils. In many formulations, three will be all that is needed. The total number of drops of a combined mixture of essential oils should range from six to forty drops.

Use the following guidelines as a rough meter to gauge by:

For mild formulations: Make the formula with six to fifteen drops. Although not an ironclad rule, try to mix a middle note oil in with any of the other two to make the solution more balanced.

For moderate formulations: Make the formula with fifteen to twenty-five drops.

For very intense and powerful formulations: Make the formula with twenty-five to forty drops.

For extra long hair: Add one more ounce of base oil, do NOT add additional drops of essential oils.

For the Scalp

Remember that the solution will be massaged deeply into the scalp and left on for several minutes. Most of the formulations will tingle, and that is OK. Check with the client to make sure it is not a "burning sensation." Once the time is up, thorough rinsing is very important.

For a mild condition or tender scalp: your essential oil mixture should be comprised of up to six total drops of oil. And leave it on for two to five minutes.

For a moderate condition: the essential oil blend should be comprised of a total of ten drops of oil. Leave it on for five to ten minutes.

Skin Care Formulas: General Guidelines

> **NOTE**
> When creating any formula, always keep in mind and/or review the previous sections detailing the characteristics of essential oils, "note" categories, and carrier/base oils.

Consult with your client while assessing the skin's general condition. Note any areas of sensitivity. Discuss your findings with the client, obtaining the most accurate information that will assist you in preparing the proper formula.

For skin care, the practitioner will be massaging the solution directly into the skin. And it will stay in the tissue for hours, if not days. The penetration ability of essential oil is why it is so effective. In ranking the three areas of the professional market—hair, skin, and nail care—aromatherapy was best designed for the skin. Essential oils travel through the epidermal tissue with ease due to their minute molecular structure, and their compatibility to the cell structure in the epidermal layers. Another element to the success of essential oils' ability to penetrate the skin is that they are lipophilic. This means that they have an affinity for fat cells. Since fat cells of the skin are found in the subcutaneous layer, the absorption rate of most essential oils is immediate.

For all cleansers you begin with a base: two ounces for each client. Add the essential oils into the base.

For sensitive skin and/or mild solutions: the mixture should be comprised of up to ten drops of essential oils. Use less top note oils.

For moderate solutions: the mixture should be comprised of up to twenty drops of essential oils. You have more freedom in selecting the various potent oils.

For powerful solutions: mix up to thirty drops of essential oils. Using the strongest top note oils may mean that the number of drops is drastically reduced. ALWAYS REMEMBER THAT LESS IS BETTER.

Nail Care Formulas: General Guidelines

Assess your client's nails and hands to determine their condition and subsequent choice of formula to use. Discuss any preliminary findings and options with the client.

In nail care, some of the work will require that the solutions be soaked in, while others will be directly massaged into the cuticle tissue, nail beds, hands and feet. For a full day's supply of an all-purpose massage oil: start with eight ounces of any base oil and add: a total of three tablespoons of three essential oils, one ounce of each.

For a single application, begin with one teaspoon of the base oil and add any one of the essential oils to it. The total number of drops should fall into the 6–10 drops range. An exception is for fighting fungi; see the listed formulas in Part II, chapters 9 and 10, to judge those differently.

Chapter 4

Contraindications to the Use of Essential Oils

*The professional esthetician must take a thorough medical history, including any known allergies and sensitivities, **before** any service is rendered. Check each of the formulations listed in this book for the information regarding the negative reactions for each. Use this information as a guide to help with the customized solutions that you create for all hair, scalp, skin, nails, pedicures, and general massage formulas.*

Hair and Scalp Care Contraindications

Hair strands will not have actual allergic reactions to any substance. Direct contact of the essential oil to the hair is limited. The formula will be made up of a neutral shampoo that ultimately will be rinsed thoroughly out of the hair.

The only slight area of concern would be if the hair was heavily chemically treated, such as being bleached blonde or a full head of weaved highlights. Some essential oils have a strong color transfer, like carrot oil. Care should be taken to avoid changing the client's hair color. There are no known ways to remove the change, since the molecular size of essential oils is so small, it does not come out as easily as it goes in.

Negative reactions can arise when using essential oils for scalp treatments. Again, it is recommended that the solution be made up of a neutral-base shampoo. Typically, the solution is massaged into the scalp and left on for several minutes, but then thoroughly rinsed out. The normal and expected reaction is for it to tingle.

First, stay by the side of the client for as long as the solution is on their scalp. Do NOT leave the client alone to fend for themselves.

Do NOT ask "Does this burn or sting?" That encourages negative thoughts and stronger reactions. Instead, ask the client how it feels. The client may describe a tingly sensation.

Second, explain that the tingle is ok, but instruct the client to immediately report if it becomes more severe. Burning or stinging sensations are signs that must be acknowledged and dealt with immediately.

If the client does comment that their scalp feels like it's on fire, immediately rinse with a mild stream of ice cold water. Do not use a full pressurized stream, as the force of the water can add to the negative reaction. While the client's head is still in the bowl, gently check the scalp for redness.

If the scalp is considerably red, make up an aloe vera gel and ice water solution of one-half ounce ice water to one ounce of aloe vera gel. Stir and **gently** pat into the scalp. Leave it on for three minutes. Then rinse for two full minutes with cold water.

With the scalp being so sensitized, do not complete a color tint, or any chemical service, afterwards. If necessary, reschedule the client for those services three days later. Do not pull on the hair. Any hairstyle requiring a lot of teasing should be put off to another day, too. Ideally, it would be best to use a hooded hair dryer on "cool setting" to dry the client's hair and postpone any other services to a future appointment. Use your best judgement in handling clients and their needs.

Common sense would also dicate that first-time scalp treatments not be provided on days that are set up for special events, such as weddings, anniversaries, or birthday parties.

Facial Skin Care Contraindications

Since you will be potentially dealing with the skin of so many different people, the chances and varieties of having a reaction are almost endless.

Sneezing

One of the more typical reactions is for the client to start sneezing. Unfortunately this is quite a problem, since their eyes, ears, throat, and nose are all connected. Sneezing indicates an internal reaction to the aroma, and the best advice is not to panic. You cannot remove the essential oil's aroma from the room immediately. It is important to improve the ventilation of the room. The best remedy would be to open a window and get a lot of fresh air to come in. For most salons, this is not a possibility. The second choice is to have an excellent circulation system, built in to the ceiling and walls. The third, and probably the most used approach, is to use two occilating fans to push the inner room air out, and pull the nonaromatic air from the outside, in.

While this is going on, have a clean, unscented towel gently wrapped over the client's face to allow for breathing. Combining the filtering of the air, and their airway, should eliminate the sneezing fairly quickly.

It would be a misconception to think that all aromatherapy treatments have to have strong aromas. Most do, however, as the professional gets more experience and training, they will learn how to mix oils that will have very mild fragrances. Some can be so light they go almost undetected.

Rashes and Hives

The reaction that causes the most concern, and rightfully so, is the rash or hive reaction. This indicates an internal release of histamine from the adrenal system and once it is triggered, it cannot be immediately neutralized without presciption medication. This does not mean that the esthetician does not have some control over the situation. **ABOVE ALL ELSE DO NOT PANIC!** The client is already experiencing some discomfort, and the level varies by each individual. They do not need to sense that the esthetician is panicking.

First, if any residue still remains on the skin, remove it immediately with very cold water and fresh, sterile cotton pads. If facial sponges were used in the early stages of the facial, put them aside and do not use them again. They will have microscopic drops of the essential oils in them. Using fresh cotton pads avoids reintroducing the irritant to the skin.

Second, it is always good to have an "allergy emergency kit" in the facial room or salon. The kit is comprised of distilled water, a wooden spatula, one sterile fan brush, a roll of cotton, a package of cotton squares, and one box of baking soda. The goal is to make a paste from the water and baking soda to be the thickness of homemade jam. Paint it over the irritated area, and then apply a sheet of cotton soaked in ice water to make a mummy wrap. Leave the paste and cotton pack on for five to eight minutes. Check the skin every three minutes. Remoisten the cotton with the ice water to maintain the coldness against the rash and/or hives. Roll the cotton wrap off of the face, taking as much of the paste as possible along with the cotton. The less wiping against the irritated skin, the better.

The third step is to acknowledge the situation in a clear, calm manner. This is not a reaction that anyone can pretend is not happening. Explain that care was taken to avoid such an experience, (avoid negative expressions, like "these hives," "this rash," or "this allergic reaction.") Remind the client that plants and herbs can effect us all. As long as a proper evaluation was done in the beginning, a clear log of all *known* allergens would have been recorded. Those elements would have been avoided. You will now add this to the client's record. One reason you can offer to the client is that perhaps the essential oil that was used has some connection to one of the known allergens. For instance, the essential oil used could come from the same plant family. It is somewhat like comparing similar characteristics of cousins. They have different parents, but they also follow a certain gene pool. A similar connection to the essential oils could be the cause of the reaction to the skin.

It is a common practice not to charge for a service during which an allergic reaction does occur. In states like California, where the atmosphere for taking legal action against others is quite high, having the policy of not charging a client turns into a high asset in court. Part of the legal system will determine if the esthetician gained financially by the action. Not charging a fee at the time of the incident shows good faith, and the courts tend to rule good faith in favor of the business.

Follow up the allergic reaction by calling the client later that day to check how they are feeling, and again in two days. If the client's skin does not return back to normal in the two days, a doctor's visit may be required. If this is a long-standing client, it would be a good gesture to cover part, if not all, of the cost of the visit. If the esthetician can show that they behaved professionally and followed up with phone calls and the offering of shared medical bills, it might reflect favorably in court. (Before offering any services, check with a competent lawyer on your options and expectations concerning possible situations. While you want to be accountable and professional, you also do not want to inadvertently open yourself to negligence.)

As mentioned in the hair and scalp care section, new essential oil facial treatments may not be the best choice for first-time clients, if they are coming in on their wedding day, special birthday, or anniversary.

Nail and Basic Skin Care Contraindications

There are two different areas of consideration in the nail department. The nails on the hands and feet will probably never cause concern in allergic reactions. The skin underneath might. Also the skin on the hands, feet, arms, and legs can be as sensitive as the skin on the face. All the precautions and remedies for facial skin apply here.

Part 2

Formulas and Recipes

Chapter 5

Hair Care Formulas and Recipes

This section is the area that will be used repeatedly by the beauty professional. It is divided into each of the specialized professional categories: hair, skin, and nails. So as to make it easier for all of the beauty technicians to use the book on a daily basis, parts of the material covered is repeated within the different sections. It is believed that the hairstylist, esthetician, and manicurist would most likely prefer to go to the sections that pertain to their area of expertise, rather than having to search throughout the book for all of the information that they will need to use aromatherapy formulas on their clients.

Overview: The Importance of Hair

The phrase "my crowning glory" has referred to a person's head of hair for centuries. Here are some examples of the key importance our hair plays in our lives:

- In some men, the amount and the thickness of their hair's appearance has a direct influence on their opinion of how masculine they appear.
- It has been a complaint of millions of husbands everywhere that their wives spend too much time "fussing with their hair."
- The police will ask, "What is the color of their hair?," as one of the first identifying features, when making a positive identification of someone.
- In the social scene, people will describe each other by the appearance of their hair.

The fuss and bother spent on one's hair has been a major reason a person decides to become a professional hairstylist. It is a profession that is guaranteed to never go out of style, and never to be obsolete. Millions of dollars are spent on advertising merchandise that

51

claim to create miracles on human hair. Hundreds of companies put their monies on glitzy ad slicks to promote the cosmetic appeal of their products.

Improving Appearances

The really potent hair care treatments are only found in a professional salon. With the addition of aromatherapy to the existing salon services, the professional hairdresser can truly make a significant contribution to the improvement of their clientele's hair.

To the untrained eye, aromatherapy may seem like some sort of magic potion. The immediate change in the appearance of the hair, can, in fact, be overwhelming to the person who has suffered for so long. To them, the hairstylist will seem like a miracle worker. If the average consumer knew that the theories behind aromatherapy come to us after thousands of years of practice, then they would realize why it works so well. After all, if every breakthrough we heard about came with thousands of years of constant research and testing to improve, we would feel confident that the results we experienced were expected and NOT magic.

Combating Competition

An added benefit to bringing aromatherapy into the professional salon is that it will add to its status within the neighborhood. Just drive around the area where your salon is located, and notice how many other salons are right near yours. Competition alone forces the professional to seek ways to stay ahead of the rest. It is no longer just a fad or trend to offer more services within the same location. Diversification is an important element to staying in business. For recent graduates from beauty schools, it will be a major asset to be able to perform aromatherapy treatments. Many graduates will be looking for a job at the same time. Those who can fit into a diversified salon, will find it easier to get hired. Adding aromatherapy into their available skills, will help to counterbalance the lack of years of experience. All recent graduates must overcome this imbalance, when looking to begin their careers.

Treating Stress

All salon employees need to keep informed on what trends are occurring in the work place. Workers will make up no less than 80% of their entire clientele base. The American workers who are career-driven, are forced to finds ways to condense their busy schedules. The salon that wants to attract these workers as part of their clientele will make ways to accommodate them. These highly driven individuals will most likely store a great deal of stress inside.

Aromatherapy has several effective treatments to deal with stress. There are many different areas that aromatherapy treatments will add to the skills and expertise of the professional hairstylist. Every condition of the hair, the scalp, and lifestyle damage to both, can be improved through the use of aromatherapy essential oils. The following is just a list of the most often sought-after solutions: **alopecia**, brittle hair, chemical build-up (ie: tar and nicotine), dandruff, dry hair, itchy scalp, oily hair, over-processed/damaged hair, and sun-damaged hair. Specific, specialized formulas are detailed in the next section. Each formula has been carefully measured, based on the author's personally developed formulas.

Shampoos

One of the most often overlooked specialties in the beauty salon is a properly executed hair shampoo. For the average client, it is just the first step to the haircut that they have to come in to get. But think of a hair salon shampoo like a professional lipstick application. Both are done thousands of times by the client, but are not performed with the skill and finesse that a professional can. And the results can be significantly different. Once the hairdresser makes it a point to offer an aromatherapy hair shampooing, the client will think twice before ever considering to go anywhere else for a shampoo again.

Aromatherapy Shampoo

What is the difference between an aromatherapy shampoo and an ordinary one? The answer is multifaceted. First is the fact that the essential oils used inside of the shampoo formula are so small they can penetrate the hair follicle. Second, they have an immediate reaction to the client's olfactory nerve, through their nasal passages. Third, the essential oil travels to the scalp and engages contact with the skin and nerve endings. Fourth, essential oils have the power to stimulate and/or sedate the client's scalp.

Therefore, an aromatherapy shampooing is really more like a deep treatment of the hair follicles than just a cleansing of the client's hair. And this is just the beginning; aromatherapy can be used to bring about a series of changes in anyone's hair. Since there is more than just one kind of formula, the professional must make some decisions based on personal observations. You can easily create personalized formulations in all your aromatherapy treatments. You can create the perfect shampoo formula right in front of the client, each and every time they arrive for their appointment.

A special secret is the freedom that aromatherapy formulas offer: you will never have to be afraid of running out of the "right shampoo," because if you are out of one element, you can substitute another essential oil or make up another treatment all together. Customizing is one of the most exciting benefits of using aromatherapy in a salon. What client would even want to switch salons, when they can only get "their private formula" with you?

Seasonal Adjustments

Remember that the seasons will have a direct effect on what the client's hair will need. Aromatherapy offers you the flexibility to customize as the seasons change. In addition, clients that do a lot of traveling are faced with many climatic changes. They will love being able to come to you, to "fix" all that traveling takes out of their hair. Aromatherapy aides you in developing client retention, based on their being dependent on you for the "formula."

CAUTION

As always be sure to ask your clients about their allergy history. Anyone can be allergic to any natural substances. Careful consideration will have to be taken when working in close quarters.

Formula Ownership

Obviously, you want to keep your special formulas written down, and in a safe place. For the salon owner, it is worth noting at this time, that these formulas should be considered "salon property" and not available to "walk out of the salon," for any reason. Some of the more common mistakes/assumptions are:

1) The employee makes the formula for the client, and therefore feels that the formula belongs to them.
2) The customer is leaving the area and wants their formula to take to the new location to be given to the salon in that area.

Salon owners have to make up their own rules. Providing a polite explanation of the rules at the beginning of employment should avoid any future problems with employees. And when a client leaves the area, simply state that the formula will stay with you should they want to visit in the future. Let them know that these formulations took years of study and training and therefore you must keep your best training with you. The client will appreciate your hard work.

There are 17 vegetable bases, as listed on page 28. For the purpose of clarity and ease of following formulas, only the most popular selections will be discussed. These are: almond oil, corn oil, olive oil, and safflower oil. All are very versatile, easy to find, and reasonably priced based on their popularity. Appendix A, at the end of the book, provides a list of suppliers of essential oils and other products. These bases can also be mixed with shampoo, although not as recommended. If chosen, these would be added in the same per-drop fashion as the essential oils are done. It is recommended that only the most advanced hairstylists in aromatherapy attempt to use the bases in this manner.

Many of the 100+ essential oils are detailed in Chapter 3. For the hair care treatments shown in the following sections, the hairstylist should have the following 25 essential oils:

1. Benzoin
2. Bois de rose
3. Carrot
4. Chamomile
5. Clary sage
6. Cypress
7. Fennel
8. Frankincense
9. Geranium
10. Hyssop
11. Jasmine
12. Juniper
13. Lavender
14. Lemon
15. Marjoram
16. Neroli
17. Orange
18. Palmarosa
19. Patchouli
20. Peppermint
21. Petitgrain
22. Rose
23. Rosemary
24. Sandalwood
25. Ylang-Ylang

Preparing for an Aromatherapy Shampoo

Supplies to have on hand: two plastic 100 mL beakers and a box of wooden tongue depressors (they make wonderful disposable stirring and application tools).

An aromatherapy shampoo can be done very quickly. However, it is strongly recommended that on the initial presentation you spend an ample amount of time. Let the client relax and enjoy what will be a most unique shampooing. Let the client feel that this is a treatment to be savored and not just rushed through. (Quickies are ok . . . but wouldn't you rather be pampered, instead?)

Step I: Verbal/Written Evaluation

You will be serving the client's best interest and get the best, quickest results by getting into the habit of proper record keeping. Start a file box index. Either a 3" x 5" card file or a 5" x 7" filing system is inexpensive and very easy to keep the client's records alphabetically. Record their name, address and phone number. The date of the service. Take down pertinent information about the client's health. Since you are not a medically trained professional, the questions should be directed to general health areas. Here are some of the questions that would make your evaluation, of the client's hair, and subsequent treatment, easier:

- Does the client consider him- or herself to be in good health? (remember, you may record observations but are not allowed by law to make a diagnosis).
- Does the client smoke any form of tobacco products, cigarettes, pipe, or cigar? If so, how much is smoked a day? How long have they smoked?
- Does the client drink alcoholic beverages? If yes, how often?
- Does the client consume caffeinated beverages such as coffee, or cola drinks? If yes, how many per day?
- Does the client use large amounts of salt?

Check with the clients to find out if they are currently taking any medication. If they are, then find out what it is, for what condition it is being taken, and whether it is a recurring prescription or just a new one that will be stopped in the very near future. For example, is it hormone replacement therapy, with a recurring prescription of estrogen, or an antibiotic for just a 10-day period to handle a mild chest infection? Both would affect how you would create the formula to use.

In LARGE LETTERS record ALL known allergies to ABSOLUTELY EVERYTHING! It would be helpful if you recorded this information in RED ink or highlight it. That way it will stand out each and every time the client comes in for services.

Record the answers to all of these questions, and any others that you may feel are important, on the file card.

On each and every repeat visit you will have the opportunity to record any changes if they are present. This is called creating a "client history," and since using aromatherapy treatments helps develop long-term relationships with your clients, you will have many opportunities to keep accurate client histories.

Aromatherapy has the flexibility to fit the needs of each client, even if those needs change over time.

Step II: Hands-on Hair Evaluation

Once you have completed the verbal questionnaire, you can begin to do a manual observation of the client's hair while it is dry. Should the client come to you with hair covered with hairsprays, hair gels, or mousse, you will have to brush the hair first to try to break or remove the coating that these products produce. Remember that this evaluation will not be as accurate as it could have been if the client's hair was without the coatings.

NOTE

When setting up new client appointments, make it a standard practice to request that all new clients come into the salon on their very first visit without hairspray, gels or mousse in their hair. This policy will make it easier for the professional hairstylist to begin evaluating the condition of the client's hair, whether or not aromatherapy treatments will be offered. If you have receptionists, they should be instructed to perform this request and/or parts of the evaluation.

The professional needs to judge the strengths and weaknesses of the hair for perming choices as well as for highlighting, or coloring processes.

Begin by examining the hair by running your fingers over the dry hair. Check for texture, softness, amount of natural moisture, any signs of damage. Check the scalp, too. Do the strands of hair feel dry, or brittle, coarse, oily, or sun-damaged, chemically-damaged, or thin, to the touch? When you run a strand between your fingers, does it glide when dry or seem to catch as you move your fingers along the strand? The hairstylist can then decide how to proceed in creating the perfect aromatherapy shampoo treatment, based on the oral and manual observation.

The Record Card

Following is a sample of what a record card may include. Notice that the categories will lend themselves to the final formulation recipe. One side of the card has the answers to questions and observations, the other side has the formulation written out. Notice the card also has the reaction after the treatment was executed. The card is written in a semi-shorthand version. This is done for time-keeping and for the privacy factor. Should anyone pick up the card it will not be as apparent what information is recorded. A full description follows this sample for the reader to understand how it works:

> Ms Susan Jones 34, F/t -sec, smk:1 pack/d, 6 c. of coff/ 3 cans of d-cola. MED: B.C.Pills, ALLERGY: GRASS/POLLENS.
> Follicle: S/D, Th, Br, Tinted

This side of the card says: Susan Jones is unmarried, 34 years old, a full-time secretary, smokes 1 pack of cigarettes a day, drinks 6 cups of coffee and 3 diet colas a day. She is on birth control pills and is allergic to grass and pollens. Her hair is sun-damaged, thin, brittle and tinted.

> Formulation: 1/1/87, 1st tr:s/d, br RECIPE: Base +8 d Jojoba,
> 6 d of Primrose, 8 d of Sesame, 8 d of Lemon. 4.5 min./ Cl/R RESULTS: Imd tex improve, high sheen- B+

This side of the card says the client came in for a treatment on January 1, 1987. It was the first treatment and the area of concentration was on the sun-damage, and brittle hair conditions. The actual formula used the standard shampoo base: 2 oz. of an UNSCENTED PH balanced mild shampoo base. Added to the base was 8 drops jojoba oil, 6 drops primrose oil, 8 drops sesame oil, and 8 drops lemon oil. The formula was worked into the hair for 4.5 minutes and rinsed out with cool water. The results were immediate texture improvement, high sheen, and overall the hair was judged to be a B+ rating.

Aromatherapy Shampoo Treatment

Place the client's head securely in the shampoo bowl. Instead of beginning by reaching for the sprayer nozzle to wet the client's hair, place a hair towel inside of the bowl and fully saturate it with VERY WARM water. Spread the very wet, hot towel under the client's hair and bring it up and around to encompass the hairline. Press firmly to transfer the heat and moisture from the towel to the hair. Re-saturate the towel.

Now, depending on what information you recorded on your file card, begin to create the "right shampoo formula" on the spot, right before your client's eyes. They love to watch and it gets others interested in what you are doing, too.

Start by mixing 2 oz. of an unscented pH-balanced mild shampoo base into the beaker. This is the base you will use for all of your formulas. Any beauty supply will be able to supply you with the most generic, mild, no-frills shampoo. (You can make your own soap base, if so inclined.) Then mix various essential oils into the beaker for the finished formulation. The various kinds of conditions and recipes for each will follow this information. First, apply the formula at the hairline, working it into the hair follicles and all the way to the ends. Spend at least 3–4 minutes working the shampoo through the entire head of hair. Re-saturate the towel with very hot (but not scalding) water. Ring it out and wrap the towel around the hair while it still has the shampoo in it. Slowly count to 10. Then remove the towel. Rinse the hair as you normally would to make sure all of the suds are completely gone and the hair is clean.

Performing the shampooing process in this way, should not require a second shampooing. Remember that the molecules of the essential oils will be able to penetrate the hair completely. This makes the whole process more effective.

Aromatherapy Head Massage

Another aromatherapy treatment that works well with aromatherapy shampoo is the aromatherapy head massage. (You are not required to be an expert masseuse, to perform this service.) This treatment adds to the time it takes to get the client ready for your hair cut (or any other service). The time, however, is well spent when it can have such a powerful impact on your client's attitude and total sense of well being.

Never underestimate the "power of touch." In today's society, most people do not have or take the opportunity to set aside a few moments to get any kind of massage. This will undeniably be the most sought-after service you will offer!

There are several different ways to approach giving aromatherapy head massages. The first method creates an atmosphere where the client senses that this treatment is being specially prepared. Other clients in the salon will look on at this approach and ask about it. Most often the question is: "What is that person having done? . . ." This leads to others wanting the same service. From a marketing standpoint this approach makes a lot of sense.

Method 1—In Designated Area

Here is how the first method unfolds. The client is asked to slip into a salon-provided robe/dressing gown. Most salons have a designated area where color/tint is applied or perms are wrapped. In this area, a countertop is near the client's chair.

Preparation
The client is to fold their arms against the countertop to support their forehead. It is recommended that you have the client close their eyes. This allows them to relax and enjoy the sensations the massage will offer. The hairstylist stands to one side of the client's head.

1. The formula is in a beaker, and the hairstylist pours it into their own palm first.
2. Spreading it between both hands, the aromatherapy head massage will begin with the nape of the neck working from one side of the head to the other. The neck area and nape of the hairline is where many people hold their stress. This area will be the most sensitive spot to work on. The client may even make little moaning sounds, or comment how "good it feels." Do not rush this part of the massage. Let the client savor the sensations.
3. Slowly move your fingertips upwards, working towards the forehead/hairline. The movements should be in small,

clockwise, circular motions. Careful attention should be paid to making certain that your **nails never scrape the scalp.** This massage uses a firm pressure of the finger pads against the scalp and nails would just make tiny nicks against the skin. The aromatherapy formulas provide additional stimulation to the scalp. Remember, essential oils easily penetrate the skin.

Method 2—At the Shampoo Bowl

Another method for conducting an aromatherapy head massage is to execute it at the shampoo bowl.

1. Place a rolled towel in the shampoo bowl's headrest area. Most shampoo bowls are not very comfortable. Since part of the advantage of doing this treatment is to take away the client's stress, it is important that they are comfortable.
2. With the client's head in the shampoo bowl, begin this massage at the front of the hairline at their forehead.
3. Work from side to side and back towards the nape of the neck.

If the client has strong neck muscles, they can lift their heads up off of the headrest/towel while you manipulate the nape and neck areas. Otherwise, hold the client's head with one hand, as you work the back of their head. This is usually the favorite part of the treatment for the clients. Many will actually get goose-bumps from all the nerve endings being relaxed. Remember not to rush through this area, it will be the most enjoyable part of the treatment.

Method 3—Combination Massage/Shampoo

You can choose to perform the aromatherapy head massage alone (by itself), or use the shampoo formulation and work it into your client's scalp and back of neck. To create the personalized aromatherapy head massage solution, mix the formula right in front of the client.

Procedure
Using one of the plastic beakers, begin with 1 oz. of a base product and add the appropriate essential oils into it (various formulations are fully explained in chapter 6).

If using just the shampoo formula, start with the aromatherapy head massage first.

1. Begin as mentioned above, using the hot towel.
2. Part the hair to expose the scalp you would apply the shampoo formula to first, starting at the forehead and working towards the back of the skull and down the nape of the neck. Use firm, small, circular motions using both hands if the client is comfortable supporting their own head. Use the one-hand method if you need to hold the client's head.
3. Spend at least 3–4 minutes massaging the entire skull and nape BEFORE moving on to work the shampoo formula into the hair.
4. Proceed to follow the shampoo technique as described above.

Pay close attention to removing the shampoo from the scalp and nape. If a thin residue is left, it can cause the client to have an itchy scalp. No shampoo is meant to be left on the skin for long periods of time (over 10 minutes).

Aromatherapy treatments have many more applications than just creating a great hair shampoo or doing an extended hair massage. The true wonder of the whole concept, is in its ability to bring about changes in the body. With hair care, aromatherapy offers the professional hairstylist the opportunity to assist the client in areas that have not been made available before.

Aromatherapy treatments are powerful resources for the salon to perform the most exciting services for the health and well-being of the clientele. In the art world, it is recognized that the condition of the canvas greatly determines the beauty of the painting. In other words, the better the canvas, the more beautiful the picture. The comparison in the hair industry would be: the healthier the hair and scalp are, the more beautiful the hairstyle can be. Aromatherapy treatments assist the hairstylist in creating a more beautiful perm, highlighting, or tint.

The reason is simple: aromatherapy treatments bring about healthier, more attractive hair and scalp conditions. This will give the hairstylist the opportunity to work with better quality hair.

Chapter 6

Specific Hair Conditions and Formulas

> *All hairstylists encounter problems that their clients experience with their hair. Some of the conditions can be helped by conventional methods along with aromatherapy treatments. Some will require medical treatment and those are mentioned as well. After the specific conditions are explained, the appropriate aromatherapy treatment and formulation will be discussed.*

The Purpose of Multiple Formulas

The purpose of offering several different formulas for the same condition is NOT to confuse the reader. The author wants to share what recipes she has found to be effective, and wants to offer the opportunity to have more than just one recipe to use. As with any experienced aromatherapist, certain amounts of trial and error are necessary to develop the skill level that is required. These formulas have been created on an as-needed basis.

As your comfort and confidence level rise, your formulations will be derived from an as-needed basis, too. In examining the blends, feel free to refer to the section explaining the individual essential oils. Some of the essential oils found in these recipes will be on that list, some are less explored and will not appear. For those who choose to develop their talents in aromatherapy, no one book can be the answer to your training.

All the formulas will work for the specific hair condition type, the preference becomes most apparent in the natural fragrances that each will create. The most noticeable reactions to each recipe, based on actual reactions, are offered. Experiment to find what will work best for your clients. Please pay close attention to any known allergies your client may have, before creating the formula.

It is impossible to have an allergic reaction in the hair alone. In dealing with the client's scalp and neck or any other skin tissue, the chance for an allergic reaction is very much a concern. Also remember that the client's air passages are connected to their eyes, ears and

throat. Breathing the essences of a known allergen can bring about a
SERIOUS AND SEVERE REACTION.

NOTE

Your nose is the most powerful of all of your senses. The
olfactory nerve can register a scent once, and 25 years
later you can remember that you smelled the scent before. You may not know exactly when, but your brain
will register it. That's just one example of how incredible
the sense of smell is. Another important note to mention, is that you will also remember a smell that is unpleasant to you. Therefore, part of your success with
aromatherapy will be based on your ability to create the
fragrances that your clients will like.

NOTE

For the formulas included in his section, it is recommended that the beaker be warmed prior to using. To do
this, run hot water over the outside of the beaker, wrap a
hot towel around the beaker, or place the beaker inside a
baby bottle warmer for approximately 5 seconds.

For beginners in aromatherapy, specific formulations are provided. Readers are encouraged to copy them for their own use. For
the professional with more advanced skills in aromatherapy, the key
essential oils known to aid in the treatment are listed so that you can
create your own formulas.

CAUTION

Special care must be practiced when using specific oils.
Remember: rosemary, sage, eucalyptus, hyssop, fennel,
and tagetes (among others) are **very dangerous** to
pregnant women. Eucalyptus and lemongrass **cannot**
be used on young children. Bergamot is **very dangerous** to any client with photosensitivity.

Alopecia

Alopecia is serious hair loss over various areas of the body, NOT to be
confused with balding. Before the hairdresser jumps in with an aro-

matherapy treatment for alopecia, the client should be directed to their medical practitioner. The doctor will be able to test for a deficiency in the pituitary gland or the thyroid gland. Obviously, if a major glandular problem exists in either of these, no amount of aromatherapy will offer much relief.

In addition, there are other key problems that will contribute to severe hair loss that would need direct medical assistance. The most obvious is **chemotherapy** for cancer treatment. Aromatherapy treatments can aid in making whatever hair remains connected in the scalp to look healthier and feel better in texture, but cannot reverse or stop the side effect of hair loss during the chemotherapy sessions.

Severe mental stress can cause alopecia, and so can radiation. Always check with the client's doctor before rendering treatment, once it is disclosed that the client has any of these medical conditions/problems. Establishing a regular practice of calling a client's doctor, prior to treatment, may provide an additional benefit: The doctor's respect. In turn, some practitioners have had many successful relationships with doctor referrals of many patients. The clientele base and professional status may increase.

If you are not medically trained, you must be careful with your words, so as not to be misinterpreted as if doing a diagnosis and providing subsequent medical advice. Law suits may follow if the client feels as if that is so.

However, there is some sound advise that you can and should offer any client that comes to you with severe hair loss:

- Avoid swimming in lakes or streams that are polluted.
- Do not swim in chlorinated pools.
- Wear a swimming cap to protect the hair somewhat from the chemicals in the water, but be aware that the pulling on and off of the cap can have its own adverse reaction to the weak follicle strength that is present in alopecia.
- Eat correctly, and, if needed, visit a licensed nutritionist for general food guidelines.

It is a good idea for all hairstylists to take the time to read up on the basic food groups. Changes have been made on how many servings of each are recommended. For example: with the increase of cholesterol in red meat, fewer servings are suggested, and more servings of fresh vegetables are now recommended.

Shampooing, as well as use of heavy conditioners, too often can be key factors to bringing on a nonmedical condition of alopecia.

"More is not better" when dealing with daily hair care. Chemical products can contribute to a residue in the hair follicle that over time can contribute to alopecia.

For the hairstylist with years of returning clientele, check the density of hair of your chemically bleached hair clients. Has there been a noticeable reduction in hair volume? Don't be a contributing factor to your client's losing their hair. Subtle changes of hair loss can result from heavy weave services. It is a high-ticket item, and currently in vogue for women to request the look, but it is also a key factor in the destruction of the hair follicle.

As the professional hairstylist, design a hair cut and style that would require little maintenance to best serve the client. Being able to avoid daily shampooing, blow-dryers, curling irons, and/or hot rollers, will aid the client in controlling the alopecia.

Shampoo Formulas for Mild Alopecia

It is suggested that the client reduce hair shampooing to once a week.

Generally effective key essential oils for alopecia: bay, carrot, cedarwood, clary sage, evening primrose, jojoba, lavender, palmarosa, rosemary, sage, ylang-ylang.

Formula #1: Begin with 2 oz. of mild, unscented, pH-balanced shampoo. Add: 5 drops carrot oil, 10 drops jojoba oil, and 10 drops lavender oil. Stir briskly. VERY GENTLY work into the hair for 6 minutes and rinse thoroughly with warm water.

This formula has a light, sweet fragrance. It will appeal stronger to women than men. It works the same for either. Please note the use of a base oil, jojoba, as part of the blend. This is just one way that aromatherapy can be so very flexible and versatile.

Formula #2: Begin with 2 oz. of mild, unscented, pH-balanced shampoo. Add: 5 drops birch, 5 drops chamomile, and 5 drops cypress. Stir briskly. VERY GENTLY work into the hair for 5 minutes and rinse thoroughly with warm water.

This formula has a positive scent for more men than women. It works the same regardless of gender.

Formula #3: Begin with 2 oz. of mild, unscented, pH-balanced shampoo. Add: 7 drops calendula, 10 drops rose, and 2 drops thyme. Stir briskly. VERY GENTLY work into the hair for 4 minutes and rinse thoroughly with warm water.

This formula has a floral bouquet with a very mild tingle from the thyme. Since thyme is such a strong essential oil, and it's a top note, only a few drops if used.

Formula #4: Begin with 2 oz. of mild, unscented, pH-balanced shampoo. Add: 4 drops bay, 4 drops cedarwood, and 2 drops clary sage. Stir briskly. VERY GENTLY work into the hair for 4 minutes and rinse thoroughly with warm water.

This has a nice woodsy fragrance that men really like.

Formula #5: Begin with 2 oz. of mild, unscented, pH-balanced shampoo. Add: 2 drops rosemary and 9 drops ylang-ylang. Stir briskly. VERY GENTLY work into the hair for 4 minutes and rinse thoroughly with warm water.

Ylang-ylang gives this formula an oriental fragrance.

Formula for Severe Alopecia/Hair Loss

(After consulting with a doctor to get their permission to conduct any treatment.)

Formula #1: Begin with 2 oz. of mild, unscented, pH-balanced shampoo. Add: 15 drops birch, 6 drops sage, and 15 drops yarrow. Stir briskly. VERY GENTLY work into the hair for 10 minutes and rinse thoroughly with warm water.

For clients who love to be outdoors, they love the fragrance this formula offers. Although sage is a top note and most often not used in large quanities, it is the condition that determines the overall formulation. Working on hair follicles is less restrictive than working on the scalp or body skin.

Brittle Hair

Brittle hair is dry hair that breaks off easily. The hair strength is badly compromised. Brittle hair is a condition usually brought on by mistreatment of the hair—either caused by the client or the professional. Abusing the hair with excessively hot utensils, such as blow-dryers and hot curlers, perms, and hair dyes can create it. If any of these are the cause, the solutions are obvious even though not always easy to follow.

However there are people who have brittle hair for other reasons. The amount of water in the hair follicle is the main factor giving hair a better look and texture.

Another cause of brittle hair is when nutrients in the root of the hair underneath the scalp are not being properly distributed. It is a common belief that any hair ¼-inch past the scalp line is totally dead. This is not altogether true. While most of the cellular activity is under the scalp and up to the ¼-inch past the scalp, the rest of the hair has the ability to absorb water and other essential oils. Cellular transfer takes place on a daily basis, whether we are aware of it or not. Only once our bodies are totally dead, does the activity level finally stop.

As a professional hairstylist, you can offer advice to your client to make some lifestyle changes. These changes may help them to reduce the internal causes of their brittle hair. Suggest to your clients to:

- Increase their water intake to at least 6 glasses of water a day (8 is best).
- Reduce their salt intake, by not adding any salt to the foods they eat. There are plenty of sources of salt in the pre-made foods they eat every day. Select salt-free choices, like sodium-free sodas.
- Eat a well balanced, high vitamin enriched diet. If they smoke, suggest that they stop altogether or at least significantly cut down. Reduce exposure to secondhand smoke to as close to zero as possible.

The professional hairstylist will find the aromatherapy treatments highly successful in reversing the brittle hair condition at the time of the treatment. The client must be put on a maintenance schedule based largely on how successful they will be in doing the above-mentioned lifestyle changes.

Shampoo Formulas for Brittle Hair

Generally effective key essential oils for brittle hair: almond, avocado, birch, calendula, carrot, chamomile, clary sage, cocoa butter, eucalyptus, evening primrose, geranium, jojoba, lavender, lemon, parsley, peach, rosemary, sandalwood, sesame, sunflower, thyme, yarrow.

Remember that all these formulas will work for the specific hair condition type, the preference becomes most apparent in the natural fragrances that each will create. The most noticeable reactions to each recipe, based on actual reactions, are given. Experiment to find what will work best for your clients.

Formula #1: Begin with 2 oz. of mild, unscented, pH-balanced shampoo. Add: 8 drops jojoba, 6 drops primrose, 8 drops sesame, and

8 drops lemon. Stir briskly. Then work into the hair for 6 minutes and rinse thoroughly with warm water.

This formula brings to the hair the shine and gloss it had lost. Clients like the fresh, light citrus fragrance. This formula uses two base oils, jojoba and sesame, that offer additional flexibility to use two top notes, primrose and lemon. The lemon oil is a top note that has less restrictions on it than other top notes.

Formula #2: Begin with 2 oz. of mild, unscented, pH-balanced shampoo. Add: 2 drops carrot, 5 drops eucalyptus, and 8 drops sesame. Stir briskly. Then work into the hair for 6 minutes and rinse thoroughly with warm water.

The eucalyptus will make the hair squeaky clean. Its natural fragrance will add to the sense of clean.

Formula for Severely Brittle Hair

Formula #3: Begin with 2 oz. of mild, unscented, pH-balanced shampoo. Add: 8 drops jojoba, 8 drops of lemon juice, and 8 drops sesame. Stir briskly. Then work into the hair for 10 minutes and rinse thoroughly with warm water.

This formula works very quickly on restoring vitality to the hair, it is also great for clients who prefer little or no fragrance in their shampoo. This formulation uses two base oils with a nonessential oil, but the juice can also be used effectively. This is just another fine example of the flexibility and versatility of aromatherapy.

Chemical Buildup

The most recognized culprit is tar and nicotine from cigarette smoke. The obvious solution is to stop smoking. Since this is a lot easier to write than it is to get the client to do so, you can offer aromatherapy treatments that will aid in the removal of the resins but NOT correct the problem. Do suggest to the client who refuses to stop smoking altogether, that a reduced tar and nicotine cigarette would be preferred. Chemical buildup from radiation or chemotherapy is difficult to remove, but over time will diminish as the treatment comes to a close. Aromatherapy can aide in the improved appearance of the hair during and after the medical treatment. It can NOT stop the chemical buildup.

Another area in chemical buildup is actually caused by the current trend in hairstyling. This is from all the gels, sprays, mousses, and other styling tools that stay in the hair after daily repeated usage. It was briefly mentioned in the aromatherapy shampoo section.

We are all looking for ways to cut down our time spent in getting ready for work. To meet that demand, manufacturers have created styling products that dry very quickly and leave the hair "in place" so that the style will stay all day. These products form a strong coating on the hair follicle and it is not that easy to shampoo and rinse out. The hairstylist has the opportunity to offer an aromatherapy treatment to remove all of these heavy residues from the client's hair.

Offering monthly "chemical buildup removal" service, will get you a very happy and loyal client. This service will help you create better styles for the client, because their hair will be in better condition. Remember the better the canvas, the more beautiful the picture.

Shampoo Formula for Chemical Buildup

Mix 1 quart of apple cider vinegar with: 3 drops cypress and 15 drops lemon oil. Let the client recline in the shampoo bowl, while this solution is rinsed over their clean, wet hair. Leave on for 5–10 minutes. Rinse with cool water.

Dandruff

Depending on the severity of the condition, it is advisable to suggest the client first seek medical attention. Strong itchy sensations, redness, edemas, open sores from picking and/or scratching, are all indicators that medical attention is the first place to start treatment. For the mild dandruff condition, the professional hairstylist can easily treat it. The main symptom: dry flaky pieces that show up in the hair and on the client's clothes. Most would see this as an indication that the hair and scalp are dry. This is not true!

Dandruff is a condition caused directly on top of the scalp. Underneath the scalp line, the sebaceous glands (oil glands) are actually over active. Then the scalp is too thick with skin cells that pile up and stick together, making it impossible for the oil sludge to come through the hair follicle/pore. The scalp gets tight, after so much cellular buildup. The scalp tries to purge itself of the cells by forcing them to detach and fall off. The client must be made aware of the tight scalp and taught how to properly massage the scalp to ease this condition.

Massaging the scalp will also help in dislodging the buildup of the dead cells more efficiently. Special shampoos can help in clearing this bothersome condition. The aromatherapy treatment shampoos can offer continual assistance in maintaining a freedom from flakes. The aromatherapy scalp treatment should be performed, at least twice, in the beginning of dealing with the mild dandruff condition. Refer to the beginning of this section, to determine if the doctor should be consulted first and then follow up with aromatherapy treatments.

Shampoo Formula for Dandruff

Formula #1: In a pre-warmed beaker, mix 2 oz. apple cider vinegar, 3 drops tea tree, 3 drops peppermint, and 1 drop benzoin. Stir briskly and massage into the scalp. Leave on for 10 minutes. Rinse thoroughly. Then, shampoo as usual.

Formula #2: In a pre-warmed beaker, mix 2 oz. witch hazel with ½ oz. lemon juice and add 6 drops eucalyptus and 1 drop tagetes. Stir. Massage into scalp. Leave on for 8–10 minutes. Rinse thoroughly. Then, shampoo as usual.

Dry Hair

There are two different classifications that make up the condition of dry hair. The most often referred to condition is when the hair is water dry. The other is when the hair is lacking in oil and is oil-deficient. Water-dry hair is directly responding to the amount of water that the client is drinking on a daily basis. A fact of nature is that the planet is made up of 70% water. The human body also needs to maintain a 70% water concentration for it to be totally balanced in nature.

Many different reasons contribute to this daily battle to maintain the balance. The brain has two rules it never breaks:

Rule #1: Above all else, keep this body alive.

Rule #2: When in doubt, refer to rule number one!

With all levity aside, the body needs water to keep the eyes from going blind, the lungs to keep pumping oxygen, the heart to pump the blood . . . you get the picture. Nowhere in the body is water not needed. Therefore, if the brain detects a lack of this vital fluid, it must make a decision, following Rule #1, where can there be less water than optimum that will NOT cause major breakdown and death?. . . . The answer is the hair, skin, and nails. Without water these three parts of the anatomy will not look or feel great, but they will not cause major destruction of body organs or death.

The client needs to drink at least 64 oz. of water per day. Juice, soups, soft drinks and coffee/tea do contribute (though anything with caffeine acts as a diuretic). But water by itself is best. Suggest to your clients that they increase their consumption of water and decrease their consumption of caffeinated coffee, teas, sodas and liquor beverages. As a professional hairstylist, you can provide instant improvement through aromatherapy treatments. Your client can do them at home, too.

For hair that is oil-deficient, aromatherapy treatments are the greatest source of the solution to the problem, since all essential oils are molecularly small enough to penetrate the stratum corneum layer, the top layer of all of the skin on our bodies. This includes the scalp and the hair follicles.

Shampoo Formulas for Dry Hair

Generally effective essential oils for dry hair: almond, avocado, birch, carrot, chamomile, cocoa butter, evening primrose, geranium, jojoba, lavender, parsley, peach, rosemary, sandalwood, sesame, sunflower, yarrow.

Formula #1: Begin with 2 oz. of mild, unscented, pH-balanced shampoo. Add: 2 drops chamomile, 4 drops jojoba, and 3 drops rosemary. Stir briskly. Now it's ready to be applied directly to the pre-wet hair. Work mixture into the hair for 5 minutes. Rinse well with cool water.

The hair restores so nicely it shines. The fragrance is so light it is barely there. Using a base oil in the blend, balances the use of an extra drop of a more powerful essential oil, like rosemary.

Formula #2: Begin with 2 oz. of mild, unscented, pH-balanced shampoo. Add: 5 drops carrot, 5 drops jojoba , 15 drops peach, and 2 drops sandalwood. Stir briskly. Now it's ready to be applied directly to the pre-wet hair. Work mixture into the hair for 5–6 minutes. Rinse well with cool water.

The peach oil makes it almost yummy to the nose—but do not try to eat it! Young clients love this formula. This formula predominately uses base oils with just a tiny touch of essential oils. Base oils can be effective treatments without essential oils added.

Formula #3: Begin with 2 oz. of mild, unscented, pH-balanced shampoo. Add: 4 drops birch, 4 drops geranium, and 2 drops lavender. Stir briskly. Now it's ready to be applied directly to the pre-wet hair. Work mixture into the hair for 5–6 minutes. Rinse well with cool water.

The geranium makes this a tremendous hit. This blend makes the hair glisten.

Formula #4: Begin with 2 oz. of mild, unscented, pH-balanced shampoo. Add: 5 drops parsley, 8 drops yarrow and 3 drops birch. Stir briskly. Now it's ready to be applied directly to the pre-wet hair. Work mixture into the hair for 5 minutes. Rinse well with cool water.

This unusual blend of essential oils has clients loving or disliking it a lot. If necessary, you can add a few more drops of parsley to neutralize the pungency of the yarrow-birch aroma. If you let the sense of smell be the only consideration for making a blend, you will find yourself limited to what help you can offer your clientele.

Shampoo Formulas for Severely Dry Hair

Formula #1: Begin with 2 oz. of mild, unscented, pH-balanced shampoo. Add: 10 drops birch, 10 drops rosemary, and 10 drops yarrow. Stir briskly. Now it's ready to be applied directly to the pre-wet hair. Work mixture into the hair for 8 minutes. Rinse well with cool water.

This will seem like a miracle transformation on the very first shampoo. The woodsy fragrance has a strong appeal for lovers of the outdoors.

Formula #2: Begin with 2 oz. of mild, unscented, pH-balanced shampoo. Add: 4 drops almond, 4 drops sunflower, and 4 drops avocado. Stir briskly. Now it's ready to be applied directly to the pre-wet hair. Work mixture into the hair for 5 minutes. Rinse well with cool water.

If glossy, shiny hair is what your client has always wanted, this formula will fulfill their request.

Formula #3: Begin with 2 oz. of mild, unscented, pH-balanced shampoo. Add: 4 drops sesame, 4 drops evening primrose, and 10 drops cocoa butter. Stir briskly. Now it's ready to be applied directly to the pre-wet hair. Work mixture into the hair for 5 minutes. Rinse well with cool water.

The cocoa butter will make some clients feel that their hair needs another rinsing. But the hair really needs the moisture.

Itchy Scalp

Refer back to the dandruff section. If this is a symptom of severe dandruff, it is best to get the client to see their doctor first. A side effect of many medications can be an itchy scalp. Antibiotics are just some of the many medications with this side effect. Most people will be on a medication of this type for a brief period of time, and then the itchy scalp will stop when the medication is stopped. During the time the client is medicated, you should consult their doctor for approval, and then proceed to offer an aromatherapy scalp treatment. The results are usually immediate.

If the scalp is very dry, it can become itchy. This can be brought about by a lack of daily water intake. Again, advise the client of the importance of drinking 64 oz. of water a day and offer an aromatherapy scalp treatment.

Shampoo Formulas for Itchy Scalp

Remember to have clients check with their doctors before proceeding with any treatments for this condition.

Generally effective essential oils for itchy scalp: benzoin, eucalyptus, peppermint, tea tree.

Formula #1: Begin with 2 oz. of mild, unscented, pH-balanced shampoo. Add: 10 drops eucalyptus. Stir briskly. Work mixture into the scalp for 7 minutes and rinse thoroughly with warm water.

This will cause the scalp to tingle a lot. This formulation is unusual in that it uses a rather high concentration of a powerful essential oil. The condition calls for strong measures in treatment. Pay close attention to the client's scalp. If it becomes too stimulated, rinse the solution off sooner than seven minutes.

Formula #2: Begin with 2 oz. of mild, unscented, pH-balanced shampoo. Add: 10 drops peppermint. Stir briskly. Work mixture into the scalp for 7 minutes and rinse thoroughly with warm water.

This formulation is another tingler! And the same precautions and observations should be used as in Formula #1 above.

Oily Hair

This condition is caused by overactive sebaceous glands (oil glands). It is usually hereditary, coming from parents with overactive oil glands. Lifestyles can bring forth this condition. The old cliches "we are what we eat" and "what goes in must come out" can best describe how lifestyle choices effect the amount of oil in our hair. A person who intakes a high level of deep-fried food will have more oil to contend with.

If the client puts a heavy conditioner full of animal fats into their scalp, it will make the hair oily. Pomades, gels and other styling products can contribute to the level of oil in the hair. Washing the hair too often, and with too harsh chemical formulas will cause the brain to attempt to bring the balance back by sending the signal for the sebaceous glands to go into high production, thus creating oily hair. The professional hairstylist can work with the client to reverse this condition. Without the client's participation, the hairstylist can only reduce the condition, not stop it.

Shampoo Formulas for Oily Hair

Generally effective essential oils for oily hair: basil, birch, borage seed, cedarwood, cypress, eucalyptus, evening primrose, lavender, lemon, lemongrass, parsley, peach, peppermint, rosemary, sage, sesame, thyme, yarrow.

Formula #1: Begin with 2 oz. of mild, unscented, pH-balanced shampoo. Add: 3 drops cedarwood, 3 drops lemongrass, 1 drop rosemary, and 2 drops sage. Stir briskly. Now it's ready to be applied directly to the pre-wet hair. Work mixture into the hair for 5 minutes. Rinse with warm water.

Woodsy, yet powerful, makes this perfect for any business executive. It can be an irritant—USE CARE. This formula is a good example of how powerful the blend can be, it uses three top notes— lemongrass, rosemary and sage—but in small quantities. This way their individual healing properties can be utilized without being overwhelming.

Formula #2: Begin with 2 oz. of mild, unscented, pH-balanced shampoo. Add: 5 drops cypress, 5 drops lemon, 5 drops yarrow. Stir briskly. Work mixture into the hair for 3–4 minutes and rinse with very warm water.

A blend of oriental with woodsy makes for an unique experience. The even distribution of power in the amount of oil used maximizes their strengths in healing the condition.

Formula #3: Begin with 2 oz. of mild, unscented, pH-balanced shampoo. Add: 2 drops basil, 12 drops lavender, 3 drops cypress. Stir briskly. Work mixture into the hair for 3–4 minutes and rinse with warm water.

Lavender lends a light fragrance which makes it very popular with many people.

Caution: Basil is the key ingredient to use with care.

This formula has a tiny amount and should not be much of a problem. An area of confusion in aromatherapy often comes in the use of herbs that are regularly used in food recipes. Basil is a fine example. Basil leaves are placed in cooking water for taste, but alway removed before eating. It is a powerful herb that has many fine properties, but must also be used carefully.

Formula #4: Begin with 2 oz. of mild, unscented, pH-balanced shampoo. Add: 7 drops peppermint, 4 drops rosemary, 6 drops thyme. Stir briskly. Work mixture into the hair for 3–4 minutes and rinse with warm water.

The peppermint and thyme will make the client's nose tingle. But the hair has no direct feelings. If the solution rests on the scalp, it will cause tingling.

Formula for Severely Oily Hair

Formula #1: Begin with 2 oz. of mild, unscented, pH-balanced shampoo. Add: 12 drops cypress, 12 drops eucalyptus, and 12 drops sage. Stir briskly. Work mixture into the hair for 7 minutes and rinse thoroughly with warm water.

The eucalyptus will cause tingling as in Formula #4 above. Sage is extremely powerful and makes this formula quick to react. Discretion needs to be considered. On one hand you want an effective solution, on the other you have to use care.

Over-processed/Damaged Hair

Over-damaged hair is probably the most frustrating condition for the professional hairstylist. In reality, certain processes done in the salon today cause the hair to become damaged. Perms, highlights, tints, blow-drying, and other utensils used to create beautiful hair styles can all damage hair.

The professional hairstylist can keep the client on a tight schedule for haircuts, offer before and after processing, and perform hair conditioning treatments to minimize the damage. They can suggest alternating the processing solutions, whenever possible. Selecting different methods to do the services will give the hair a break from over-processing.

Aromatherapy treatments are particularly successful due to the molecular size and ease of entry into the hair follicle. Damaged hair is most often very porous, thus making the entry easier.

There are other lifestyle choices that also damage the hair: excessive drinking of alcoholic beverages, and smoking cigarettes, pipes, cigars, or marijuana. Medical treatments like **radiation**, and chemotherapy also damage hair. Common sense tells us to refer all of these reasons to a medical practitioner. Reducing the drinking and smoking makes sense, but the client may not want to hear this advice from you. The practitioner must take care in not overstepping the boundaries of the relationship with the client. Advise from a doctor or family member is sometimes better received than when it comes from the hairstylist.

Aromatherapy will provide immediate, temporary results, for the client who continues to follow a heavy usage of drinking and smoking.

Shampoo Formulas for Over-processed/Damaged Hair

As mentioned above, this really is an area that can cause a dilemma for the professional hairstylist. Offering pre- and post-treatments may be the only solution.

Generally effective essential oils for over-processed/damaged hair: carrot, eucalyptus, evening primrose, jojoba, lemon, lemon juice, sesame.

Formula #1: Begin with 2 oz. of mild, unscented, pH-balanced shampoo. Add: 6 drops evening primrose, 8 drops jojoba, and 8 drops sesame. Stir briskly. Work mixture into the hair for 5 minutes and rinse thoroughly with warm water.

Repairing the damage cannot happen overnight. With repeat usage, this formula will give the hair a second chance. This is another example of the use of base oils as the primary element of the formulation.

Formula #2: Begin with 2 oz. of mild, unscented, pH-balanced shampoo. Add: 2 drops carrot, 8 drops lemon, and 8 drops sesame. Stir briskly. Work mixture into the hair for 5 minutes and rinse with warm water.

The lemon makes it fresh, the sesame improves the shine. This has broad appeal.

Formula for Severely Over-processed/Damaged Hair

Formula #1: Begin with 2 oz. of mild, unscented, pH-balanced shampoo. Add: 5 drops eucalyptus, 8 drops jojoba, 8 drops lemon, and 8 drops sesame. Stir briskly. Work mixture into the hair AND SCALP for 4 minutes. Put a plastic cap on head, place client under a warm dryer for 5 minutes. Then thoroughly rinse with warm water.

Perky and tingly is how the client will remember this shampoo-ing. Again, two base oils allow the use of two powerful top note essential oils in the same formula with terrific results.

Sun-damaged Hair

"Prevention is worth a pound of cure" is an old cliche that fits this condition. The obvious is to wear protective garments when out in the sun. Sunscreen can be applied to the scalp and hair, but because it will make the hair appear oily, and ruin the appearance of a fresh, clean hairstyle, it is likely not going to be an effective solution. The client won't want to do something that will make them look less at-tractive.

Most outdoor activities are based around social fun. Therefore, the client wants to look their best. The professional hairstylist can suggest moderation, limiting the sun exposure to before 10 A.M. and after 2 P.M. The sun's rays are most damaging then. But most often, the professional can just be there to offer an aromatherapy treatment after the day-in-the-sun is finished. During the summer months, it would be advisable to put the active outdoorsman on a tight sched-ule of maintenance of post-sun treatments.

Shampoo Formulas for Sun-damaged Hair

As stated earlier, the best solution is to protect the hair from the sun. If that is not possible, than the professional hairstylist can offer aro-matherapy treatments.

Generally effective essential oils for sun-damaged hair: car-rot, eucalyptus, evening primrose, jojoba, lemon, lemon juice, sesame.

Formula #1: Begin with 2 oz. of mild, unscented, pH-balanced shampoo. Add: 8 drops lemon, 8 drops sesame, and 4 drops primrose. Stir briskly. Work mixture into the hair for 5 minutes and rinse with warm water.

Fresh, glossy and healthy are adjectives that the clients have used after several shampoos with this formula.

Formula #2: Begin with 2 oz. of mild, unscented, pH-balanced shampoo. Add: 2 drops carrot, 8 drops lemon, and 8 drops sesame. Stir briskly. Work mixture into the hair for 5 minutes and rinse with warm water.

This is very similar to Formula #1.

Chapter 7

Specific Skin Care Formulas and Recipes

Of all the areas within the beauty industry that can benefit from aromatherapy, the skin care area is the grandest. Aromatherapy has the largest, more powerful impact on skin care, in almost endless ways. The author's personal formulations, that have been used for more than two decades, are offered in this next section. In addition to the medicinal side of aromatherapy, skin care is what aromatherapy was designed for centuries ago.

Essential Oils and Skin Care

There are more than a thousand ways that aromatherapy has been successful, and it is most effective in the treatment of skin. In ranking the three areas of the professional market—hair, skin, and nail care—aromatherapy was best designed for the skin.

The basis for aromatherapy treatments are the essential oils. It is through their absorption, that the changes are made. The essential oil travels through the epidermal tissue with ease due to its minute molecular structure, and its compatibility to the cell structure in the epidermal layers. Essential oils are considered the inner core of all plants and roots, their heart and soul, so to speak. All the vital life force of the plants and roots are found within the molecules of a singular drop of oil. Essential oils contain the hormones of the plants and roots from which they are extracted. It is through the power of the life force of the plants and roots, that the essential oils can assist the human body's natural defenses.

This is accomplished through the essential oil's ability to limit the growth of microorganisms. Some essential oils have been able to destroy microorganisms, making these essential oils "nature's antibiotics." Essential oils have a track record of assisting the skin's defense against acne. They have a direct healing quality to human skin.

Skin is comprised of keratin fibers, and essential oils are directly absorbed in keratin. An individual molecule of a processed essential oil can be so small that it would register 710 on a **nanometer**. A human skin cell can measure 660. In layman's terms, this means that some processed essential oils are smaller than a human cell, making penetration easy.

Another element to the success of essential oils' penetration of the skin is that they are **lipophilic.** This means that they have an affinity for fat cells. Since fat cells of the skin are found in the subcutaneous layer, the absorption rate of most essential oils is immediate.

Nothing on this planet can live without oxygen. As the skin matures and ages the transfer of oxygen is challenged as various elements of the skin's fiber become weak. Through the breakdown of collagen, keratin, facial muscles, and capillaries, the passage of oxygen grows more difficult through time. The skin loses its coloring, leaving a more pallid appearance. The skin's texture becomes more grainy, and the connecting tissues begin to sag. With the aide of the oxygen within all essential oils, the skin can become revitalized.

The beneficial components of the plants and roots that make up the essential oils are offered to the skin through absorption. Essential vitamins are also given to the skin, once the essential oils penetrate the epidermal tissue. When this text discusses the skin and the effects aromatherapy has on it, the specific area of concentration are on the face, neck, and shoulders. Although we have skin all over our bodies, and most of what essential oils can do will be beneficial for all the skin on our bodies, special attention will be made to the face. After all, an esthetician's primary work area is the face, neck and shoulders.

Conditions Affecting Skin

Your face tells so much about you and your life. Wrinkles tell the passage of time, and the experiences that unfolded to get them. Frown lines mark unhappiness and stress, whereas laugh lines tell of humor and good times. The skin on our faces reveal our stress and our emotions more than any other area of our bodies. Hormonal levels are detected by the blotches or blemishes that seem to "pop up" every month. The whole world can "read us" by the appearance of our faces. And the whole world has a direct effect on our skin, too.

Climatic conditions directly affect the skin's appearance. Hot weather can produce "**heat rash**" and bumps, cold weather will produce rough, peeling, dry patches. Our environment includes lifestyle elements that also directly impact our skin and its appearance. Examples: smoking cigarettes, or dealing with secondhand smoke, smog from car fumes or factory smoke stacks and even **"acid rain."** Gone are the days when being able to wash in "rain water" was considered to be the purest, cleanest kind of water on this planet. Times have changed.

Aromatherapy can be used to successfully aid the skin in all of its battles to stay healthy, vital, and beautiful to look at as well as to touch. Remember that the seasons will have a direct effect on what the client's skin care needs. Aromatherapy offers you the flexibility to customize as the seasons change. In addition, the clients who do a lot of traveling will be faced with many climatic changes. They will love being able to come to you, to "fix" all that traveling takes out of their skin. Aromatherapy assists you in developing client retention, based on clients being dependent on you for their "formula."

The Skin and Its Functions

The skin is a natural barrier to foreign particles that try to get inside the body and hurt it. (Remember that the brain is the #1 barrier.) So the first question that would pop into your mind, might be how do we know that the essential oils can break through? The answer comes from all the extensive testing that has been conducted in research labs where essential oils have been tracked through the breath, feces, perspiration, and urine. They have been tracked into the dermis layer of the skin with the purity of the essential oils maintained.[1]

The skin has eleven different jobs to do, and the brain must keep an ongoing progress report on which jobs have been completed and which remain undone. You could relate this to the idea of having eleven different work assignments to have to get done in one day. Obviously you would have to determine which you did first and what you could put off until a later time. Eventually you would have to get to them all, but a prioritizing process would be necessary. Aromatherapy is just one successful way to help your skin keep all of its functions running smoothly. Readers will approach this subject from various levels of expertise and knowledge about the skin.

Following is a brief review of the key elements about the skin. This is not to take the place of a more detailed study guide. After much thought and consideration, this author has decided to describe how the skin works, in nontechnical terms, as she does to her personal clientele (most of whom are NOT licensed professional hairdressers, estheticians, or manicurists). It is with sincere reservations that the following prove to be of as much assistance in your needs as it has been in mine.

A Layman's View of How Skin Functions

It has been proven that you retain 10% of what you hear, 70% of what you see, and 100% of what you hear, see and can do yourself. With this in mind, the following was created to help clients form "mental images" to aide them to better understand what skin care is all about. Of particular concern was what was being done during a facial treatment, and what could be accomplished at home.

The skin weighs less than 10 pounds and is comprised of three formal layers called the **epidermis, dermis,** and **hypodermis.** The stratum corneum layer, the top layer of the epidermis, is the what we see when we look into the mirror. Although the cells are now flat, dry and fairly dead, they didn't start out that way.

The Skin as a House

It might be easier to think of the structure of the skin like the construction of a three-story house. On each floor are several rooms. Each room has its own function, such as a bedroom, bathroom, living room, or kitchen. When inside each room, you are aware of the specific function or activity that takes place. Upon reviewing the blueprint of the house, you could see that each room has support beams and floorboards and walls that are shared by the others on the same floor. To travel from one floor to the next you could use the staircase to go up and down, or perhaps an escalator that goes only in an upward direction. Though essential oils and some cosmetics can penetrate *down* into the skin, the skin itself moves only in an *upward* direction.

Consider the epidermis the top floor of this three-story house. It has five rooms, the stratum corneum being the roof. With thatched shingles, this horny layer is flat and compressed tightly to keep foreign objects, sun and wind from getting too deep inside the house. Dead skin cells are sloughed off this layer.

The dermis layer, or basal layer or otherwise called the "true skin" is the second floor of the house and it has control of all the glandular activity of the skin. All sebaceous glands (oil), sudoriferous glands (sweat), hair follicles, capillary blood supplies, and the cells are still very much alive, plump with water and vitamins. The collagen and elastin fibers are manufactured here on this level. Lymphatic glands are pumping on this level.

The bottom floor of the house is the hypodermis, commonly called the subcutaneous layer; it is the padding of the skin. Like a thick sleeping bag, it protects the skin from the bones underneath. It keeps the food supply for the activities on the first and second floor. It stores the main fibers of the nerve endings that run through the skin. Think if it as like the electrical wiring that allows you to turn lights on throughout the house. These nerve endings relay messages of pleasure and pain throughout the three layers.

The Skin—Excretory Organ

The skin is an **excretory organ.** This means that it acts like a filter to release toxins and unwanted material to the surface of the skin, the stratum corneum. The lymphatic system also deals with ridding the body of toxins and waste material.

In the human body constipation (not enough water/lubricant) and diarrhea (too much water/lubricant) are nature's way of balancing the digestive and excretory systems. Both of these conditions are used to bring about a change. The skin uses the same principles in that constipation of the skin appears as blockages, such as milia or whiteheads. Pustules and blackheads, or comedones, are the skin's form of diarrhea. One of the key roles of the esthetician is to keep the skin's moisture level balanced, so that neither condition is rendered too often.

Skin's Development: One-way Direction

The staircase and escalator refer to the passageways of the follicular channels, nerve endings, capillaries, lymph nodes, and cellular layering of the skin. The development of the skin cells is such that they travel in ONE-DIRECTION only: upward. The escalator is the example of moving steady and continually in one direction. As the escalator gets older, it doesn't function as smoothly, or quickly and from time to time might need an adjustment or two to keep it running.

The skin works on an interesting timetable. Up until the body is 25 years old, it takes cellular development 28 days to finish its journey to the stratum corneum. It takes roughly one month to go from the bottom of the dermis to the top of the epidermis. Within the next 10 years, up until around 35 years old, the same journey now takes five weeks. Add another 10 years, around 45 years old, and it then takes six weeks; at age 55 it takes seven weeks to reach the top.

As the body ages and slows down, the cellular debris increases, so the skin has more material that can get stuck on the way up. Many women get frustrated as they begin to see what they think is adolescent acne plugs on their very middle-aged skin. They ask, "How is it possible to be reliving the teenage years?" This timetable information has helped them understand the process better.

The staircase represents the ability to go into the various layers of the skin through absorption. Using aromatherapy essential oils, you can offer assistance to the various activities of the skin, where and when it is needed. The special areas of assistance will be in acne, dealing with **milia, comedones, pustules, and papules,** dry skin, oily skin, mature-lined tissue, sun damage, and wrinkles. All of these can be dealt with by treatment sessions in a salon facial room and by at-home regimens. For this book's purpose, the majority of material is directed for the facial room only.

Facials

There are many different ways to conduct a facial. This author has 76 different facials in her repertoire. She counts on providing variety to each and every client, for many reasons. One is because she hates monotony, and looks for change just to keep her own interest. Another is competition, she knows that her clients never know what facial they will receive beforehand. It keeps them interested and no one else could offer them the same facial that she offers, since no one but this author knows what it will be.

This varied program helps in inventory control. After all, since no one knows ahead of time what will be done, if you run out of one essential oil, you can just use something else. In all fairness, a standard cleansing facial should be described at this time, so that it can be compared in kind to an aromatherapy facial.

The heart of any skin care business is the facial. This section covers the methods used for a conventional facial and an aromatherapy facial. During the comparison of both, the manual method of conducting a facial is used. Electrical facials and the holistic concept behind aromatherapy are not compatible. There are many skin care specialists trying to mix the two. This approach is dangerous. The power of the essential oils are so strong that adding electricity to them is foolish and possibly seriously harmful. Even if you prefer to use electrical current during standard facials, select to do a manual facial when providing aromatherapy treatments.

Standard Manual Cleansing Facial

Products used:

Pre-bottled foamy, gel cleanser, and a makeup remover solution

Pre-bottled tonic rinse with sprayer attached

Jar of scrub/exfoliant, usually a honey-almond malt formula

Jar of clay mask—to purge and dry

Jar of gel mask—to moisturize

2–3 Jars of night creams—various thicknesses and degrees of oil concentration

2–3 Jars/vials of detoxifying serums—concentrates to be applied under the mask and before the night cream

2–3 Jars of day creams to finish the facial after the mask is removed.

Equipment used:

Facial bed/chair

Magnifying lamp—3 or 5 diopter lens

Steamer

Hot towel caddie/crockery cooking pot

Prepare your facial room/area as usual—layout of the sheets, towels, cotton squabs, etc., as customary and following state guidelines

Evaluation

You may have fifteen or more varieties of this style facial. The first basic element of any standard cleansing facial is the evaluation of the skin. You can't jump in and begin to clean if you do not have any idea what you are cleaning!

1. Clean the client's face. If the client is wearing makeup, remove all the makeup using a water soluble cleanser, or makeup remover solution.
2. Cover the client's eyes, usually with cotton pads.
3. Bring the magnifying lamp over the face.
4. Begin to inspect the skin under the light.

Evaluate the skin and check for some of the following characteristics:

- Thickness of skin
- Texture of skin
- Evenness of coloring
- Location of scars and birth marks
- Pore size
- Milia/whiteheads and comedones/blackheads
- Pustules and papules
- Any areas of irritation
- Edema
- Capillary extension/couperose
- Wrinkles
- Fine lines
- Muscle tone

The esthetician should record on the client card all aspects of this evaluation.

Informing Clients: Traditional vs. Holistic Approach

There are different ways to handle the next step of informing the client. Traditionally, during and immediately after the evaluation, the esthetician shares the findings with the client, reporting exactly how many clogged pores, wrinkles, folds, and weakened muscle control, etc., they see. The idea that clients, often female, allow themselves to undress, remove all makeup, and have a magnifying lamp put over their faces to be inspected and reviewed in this manner can be quite unsettling, leaving them feeling like their personal value of themselves is being attacked, which can lead to decreased self-esteem during the process. Even men have a difficult time hearing what is wrong with their skin.

Another approach is the holistic approach, wherein this reporting process is entirely different. Holistic medicine attempts to treat the mind and the body as one system, not exclusive of each other. A whole book could be written on this aspect alone; however, only a quick overview is provided here. Aromatherapy, in itself, is definitely a holistic practice, therefore it only makes sense to share a holistic approach to reporting the health and well being of the skin.

Part of the holistic approach deals with remembering that positive energy yields positive results and negative energy yields negative results. Telling a client what is WRONG with them, no matter how well-intentioned the messenger, the result is the same . . . the client feels bad about their skin and themselves.

To provide a comparison between the traditional and the holistic approach, the following is a hypothetical scenario describing a fictitious client with a fictitious profile. The evaluation information is exactly the same for both approaches. The difference will become clear as you read on. Most abbreviations have been left out of the evaluation to make this easier to follow.

Ms. S. Jones, 46 yrs. old, first facial ever in her life, smokes: 1 pack daily (low tar), works as a receptionist in a large office.

Medications: estrogen supplements, high-dosage vitamins/(O-T-C)

Allergies: ragweed, grass, cats (loves to garden)

Reason for visit: Birthday present

Currently uses: cleansers, day cream, eye cream (no brand preference/grocery store)

Inspection: Small scar over left eyebrow—very old, frontalis muscle lines very apparent, deep orbicularis oculi, and oris imprints, nose and chin full of large comedones (est. 400), right side of cheek and chin milia (est. 11), texture dry except mouth and nose, full capillary/couperose extension on both cheeks, more on the right side.

Traditional Approach to Client

"Ms Jones, let me tell you what I have found, I see that you have a small scar over your eyebrow, I notice some lines on your forehead, eyes and mouth areas. There are about 400 blackheads in your T-zone, that's your nose and chin area. And I count around 11 whiteheads on your right side. Your cheeks seem a little dry and I see a lot of your capillaries on your cheeks. TODAY, I am going to work on improving all that, ok?"

The esthetician really believes that should make the client happy, that they are going to get a lot of help to look better . . right? *Wrong, wrong, wrong.*

Ninety-eight percent of the time, the client doesn't even know that any of this is going on, let alone that it's something to change.

She came in because it was a gift, she does not have a clue as to what a skin care regimen is all about, let alone what a facial is.

Holistic Approach to Client

"Ms. Jones, since this is a special gift, I would like to make sure it's a memorable one. Do you have any interest in learning what my review uncovers?" (Give her the chance to say if she wants to hear it. Let's say she does, then continue.)

"The old scar on your eyebrow, did it involve a bike, like mine did?" (This lets her know that others have scars to deal with and it's ok.) "You mentioned that you garden, do you wear a hat or sun shades when you do?" (No is her answer.) "The reason I ask is that they would help you with squinting in the sunlight and not making your muscles having to work so hard." (This tells her the lines on her face are noticeable, but the focus is on a lifestyle choice—gardening without protection—which she can then decide if she wants to make a change.) "The next two questions may sound strange, and might lead you to think I'm psychic, but by any chance, Ms. Jones, are you left-handed, and do you sleep on your right side?" (She confirms she is left-handed and does sleep on her right side.)

"Let me explain why I asked, I notice that the right side of your face shows signs that you may cup the phone on your right cheek and chin, so that you can still have your hand free to write. I know that being a receptionist must keep you busy all day. The pressure of the plastic handset forces activity under the skin that shows under this magnification. Perhaps you could ask your office manager, if a head piece could be installed to free you from having to press the handset against your skin all day." (She says she did not realize that it could be affecting her skin so much.)

"And when we sleep mostly on one side, the oil glands tend to filter out onto that side, kind of like rolling down a hill. I can see on your right cheek and chin where the oil has collected. During this very first facial, I am going to be like your personal maid, and clean every nook and cranny I can during this hour. When I am finished, you'll have your 'house' as clean as I can get it in the first treatment." (There is no mention of the damage the smoking is doing to her face and skin; currently everyone is aware that smoking is bad for one's health. The client does not want to hear how bad her habit is, if she could/wanted to stop, she would. After a longer relationship is developed between the esthetician and the client, it would then be appropriate to mention that no facial can have the same results on a smoker than on a non-smoker.)

With this approach, the client's personal self-esteem stays intact, the esthetician is perceived to be a helper and one that has her best interest at heart, and with the re-telling of the information collected during the evaluation, the esthetician now knows more about her lifestyle and habits to make repeat visits more effective, too.

By mentioning that this is the first treatment, it is a subtle way to let her know that other facials should be considered. This is just one part of a soft-sell approach that can be very effective in developing a full booking.

Post-Evaluation Standard Facial Treatment

The client's skin is clean, the evaluation is complete. It has been decided that a deep cleansing facial will be executed. Specific attention will be made to the clogged pores, dry texture on the cheeks, and overall wrinkles of the face.

GOAL: To unclog the comedones around the nose, restore the moisture level to the cheeks, and soften wrinkle lines around the eyes and mouth.

Remember, no esthetician can expect to erase years of lifestyle choices and abuse in one single treatment. Setting a reasonable goal will make the client and the esthetician believe that the most was accomplished in a limited time.

Procedure

1. Steam the skin while a light cleansing massage, using the scrub/grains, is executed.
2. Remove scrub with water and sponges or cotton pads.
3. Spray skin with selected tonic.
4. Deeply massage detoxifying serum into the face, neck and shoulders.
5. Perform second massage, using a light night cream on the same areas.
6. Apply a light film of clay mask with a brush over the neck and face.

7. Remove mask with water and hot towels.
8. Respray tonic.
9. Lightly massage with selected day cream for protection.

Inform all FIRST TIME clients that any extractions are done on the second and subsequent sessions, never on the first facial. The client should be advised that an additional session should be booked and at that facial, manual extractions will be performed. Even the best, most skilled estheticians cannot guarantee that extractions won't have a negative sensation to some or all of them. When establishing a new client relationship, it is important that the client leaves having had a pleasant experience. This practice has also proven to be very succesful in getting clients to immediately book for an additional treatment.

Time Allowance

The standard time for a cleansing facial can vary. Currently, the average is 60–75 minutes, for a single-room facial operation. Most estheticians work on the "per-service" method. This means that the monies earned are generated only when they are performing a fee-paid service, as opposed to being paid by the hour, whether they work on customers or clean stock room shelves. For the estheticians who base their earnings on the per-service basis, the length of time needed to conduct the facial has a direct effect on their earning power.

In the per-service category, it is recommended that the facial last no longer than 60 minutes. Booking every 75 minutes gives you time to get the room ready for the next client, while the last one gets dressed and goes to the front desk to pay for their services and products. As the old cliche says, "Time is money and money is time-worthy."

The Positive Practitioner

Remember that aromatherapy is just one part of the holistic concept. A major characteristic of the holistic concept is positive energy fields. It would be unrealistic to think that you can walk into work, with a natural smile on your lips and twinkle in your eyes every single day of your life. Life can be challenging for all of us. The conflict arises when your clients are expecting you to be "up, positive, and happy-go-lucky" each and every time they have an appointment to see you.

It is part of why they come to you in the first place. They want to be made to feel better, and you are there to wait on them to make that happen. So on particularly challenging days, here are some tips to help get you through it:

- Count to ten backwards before you walk through the door. When you reach 1, exhale all of your oxygen, inhale deeply and smile.
- If your fingers are cold (and when you are under stress, they usually are) run them under very warm water, or hold a hot towel with both hands to get them warmed up.
- If you still feel a bit negative, vigorously shake your hands, before starting the facial.

These steps may seem odd to you at first, but they do work. Living your life with a more holistic consciousness will become a major asset for all aspects of your life. Being able to offer a more positive, up-lifting atmosphere at work will make your boss, fellow co-workers, and your clients very happy.

Aromatherapy Facial

The equipment for an aromatherapy facial can be the same as for a standard facial. Also follow the same guidelines for extraction, as mentioned in the standard first facial, above. The products used, however, are totally different.

The difference between an aromatherapy facial and a standard facial can be compared to cooking from scratch or buying a ready-to-heat frozen microwave dinner. Both have their positive points. Both have value. However, the meal prepared from scratch leaves a more positive feeling about the meal, the tastes and flavors of the food are more intense, and the general reaction from others sharing the meal are more loving. Aromatherapy facials will bond you and your client closer and more quickly than the standard facial.

Products Used*:

- Choice of 17 vegetable bases/carrier oils (refer to the list on page 28.)
- Choice of essential oil(s)

- One jar of clay powder (for a clay mask)
- One jar of aloe vera gel (for a gel mask)
- One 16 oz. cleanser base
* See formula listed in the skin care aromatherapy formulation section.

For the purpose of clarity and ease of following formulas, this text will cover the most popular selections. They are: almond oil, corn oil, olive oil, and safflower oil. For a standard aromatherapy facial treatment, the esthetician should have the following 25 essential oils:

1.	Benzoin	14.	Lemon
2.	Bois de rose	15.	Marjoram
3.	Carrot	16.	Neroli
4.	Chamomile	17.	Orange
5.	Clary sage	18.	Palmarosa
6.	Cypress	19.	Patchouli
7.	Fennel	20.	Peppermint
8.	Frankincense	21.	Petitgrain
9.	Geranium	22.	Rose
10.	Hyssop	23.	Rosemary
11.	Jasmine	24.	Sandalwood
12.	Juniper	25.	Ylang-ylang
13.	Lavender		

(Remember: Your nose is the most powerful of all of your senses. The olfactory nerve can register a scent, once and 25 years later, you can remember that you smelled the scent before. You may not know exactly when, but your brain will register it. That's just one example of how incredible the sense of smell is. An important note to mention, is that you will also remember a smell that is distasteful to you. Therefore, part of your success with aromatherapy will be based on your ability to create the fragrances that your clients will like.)

Everything in an aromatherapy facial is custom-blended on the spot for each and every client. You do not have to have a large, overstocked "back bar," because you will be creating the products as you need them, for every customer. Even if you run out of a specific essential oil, you will always be able to "pitch hit" with another selection without losing the results you were seeking. Several essential oils act similar in nature. Though their personal attributes will vary slightly, however, their reactions to the skin can be similar.

```
┌─────────────────────────────────────────────────────┐
│                      CAUTION                          │
│  As always, be sure to ask your clients about their   │
│  allergy history. Anyone can be allergic to any       │
│  natural substances. Careful consideration will have  │
│  to be taken when working in close quarters.          │
└─────────────────────────────────────────────────────┘
```

Evaluation

The steps are the following:

1. Begin the aromatherapy facial with the evaluation of the skin, just like the standard cleansing facial.
2. Next, mix the cleanser/makeup remover and clean the client's skin. Refer to the list of formulas later in this chapter.

    It would be advantageous to keep in your facial "back bar" two pre-made aromatherapy makeup removers for continual use. One for heavy makeup/resistive mascara, and the other for a light makeup cover. These two fit for every skin type. These two are pre-mixed in 6 oz. bottles. The formulas are listed on pages 99–104. (For the example of Ms. Jones' facial, Formula #1 would be used.)

3. Cover the client's eyes, usually with cotton pads.
4. Bring the magnifying lamp over the face.
5. Begin to inspect the skin under the light (review conditions and characteristics to check as previously listed on page 87–88).
6. Record evaluation information on client card.

Share your evaluation with the client, using some previously discussed holistic approaches (refer to conversation with Ms. Jones, pages 90 to 91).

Post-Evaluation Aromatherapy Facial Treatment

The client's skin is clean, the evaluation is complete. It has been decided that an aromatherapy cellular unclogging facial will be executed. Specific attention will be made to the debris in the pores, dry texture on the cheeks, and overall wrinkles of the face (the same as in the standard facial).

GOAL: To unclog the comedones around the nose, restore the moisture level to the cheeks, and soften wrinkle lines around the eyes and mouth.

Remember, no esthetician can expect to erase years of lifestyle choices and abuse in one single treatment. Setting a reasonable goal will make the client and the esthetician believe that the most was accomplished in a limited time. Notice the goal is the same for the standard facial as well as the aromatherapy one. The treatments are different, but the goals, of course, would be the same since they are based on the same evaluation.

Steam and Massage

In an aromatherapy process, the esthetician must custom blend the cleansing massage vehicle. The selected cleanser is not the same as would be in a standard facial. For this step decide which cleanser to make based on the client evaluation. Formulas for cleansers and tonics are provided later in this chapter. The formulas are numbered for ease of copying them. For Ms. Jones' facial, the cleanser selected is Formula #6, variation A. Notice that the amount of product will be only two ounces, or less. This virtually ends any product waste!

The method of massaging is the same in both approaches (standard and aromatherapy). The shoulders, décolleté area, neck, ears, and face are manipulated. Most often effleurage strokes are used. The approximate length of time for the cleansing massage and steaming is 8–10 minutes.

Procedure

1. Steam the skin while performing a light, cleansing massage.
2. Remove cleanser with distilled water and sponges.
3. Spray the skin with a tonic, using a spray bottle to provide a more even coating of the tonic. An aromatherapy tonic will work very quickly. (For the example of Ms. Jones' facial, tonic Formula #2 is used.)

Custom Recipe Massage

Creating the products to accommodate the specific goals set out during the evaluation process is the real custom work that makes this part of the facial the most exciting. You have endless recipe-creating opportunities.

For the example of Ms. Jones, you can add anti-oxidants to the moisturizing formulation to aid in the problems that her smoking has caused. Smoking has contributed to the extension of her capillaries, and you now are free to adjust the formula to include vasoconstrictors, too. To create the formula designed specifically to consider both of Ms. Jones' conditions:

Pour 1 oz. of sesame oil into a sterile beaker and add: 8 drops vitamin E (a wonderful antioxidant), 8 drops aloe vera juice, and 8 drops chamomile oil. Stir vigorously, and disburse over Ms. Jone's face, neck, shoulders and décolleté area.

Effleurage massage movements are used to help the formula penetrate. Particular attention is given to her right side where the couperose is most prevalent, and the areas around her eyes and mouth where the smoking and direct sunlight have caused the deepest wrinkles.

Noted within the lists of recipes at the end of this section, are recipes that will aide the skin of smokers. The amount of product for the formula will be under 2 oz. As the facial is continued, you will see how easy it is to keep your product usage down to the exact milliliter. (The savings in direct overhead cost makes aromatherapy facial treatments far more enticing to the business-minded esthetician.)

Once the product is made, any massage technique will work to get the product to penetrate and be absorbed into the skin. In fact, brushing the product over the skin would work, although not as well. As previously noted, the molecular size of the essential oils makes penetration a breeze. At this point, performing a deep tissue massage will add to the relaxation of the client, and at the same time reduce any stress. Apply the custom recipe.

Using your finger pads, apply slow, direct pressure beginning at the shoulders and working upwards to the forehead. Follow the facial muscles movements, using effleurage massage techniques all over them. (Massage techniques are covered in-depth in Chapter 12.) Playing melodic music while this deep tissue massage is being performed would be an added benefit. The more body senses you involve during your treatment, the more effective you will be in reducing stress in the client's body.

All essential oils provide excellent viscosity for any massage movement. After the solution penetrates, a light film should still be noticeable on the surface of the skin.

The Mask

The next product to be created is a mask. To continue this example for Ms. Jones, a clay-base mask is suggested for detoxifying the pores.

Place 1 oz. of bentonite clay in a beaker and add: 8 drops peppermint oil, 4 drops almond oil and 4 drops clary sage oil. Mix it together and spread over Ms. Jones' face. Leave on for 8 minutes.

Refer to the list of formulas (pages 116–118, 120–126 and 132) for the right recipes for your client. Again, note that only a single use is needed, so you only have to make enough to coat one face. On the average, one ounce will do.

Procedure

1. Apply formula to face, but not too close to the eyes and mouth.
2. Leave on the skin for 8–12 minutes.
3. Remove formula and residue with warm towels. (NOTE: A crock-pot or similar cooking pot, works just as well warming towels as does a "hot towel caddie." It may not look as professional, however $32 for a cooking pot versus $600 for a caddie, makes a strong argument to forego the image for the reduced costs.)
4. Respray the skin with the chosen tonic.

Day/Night Cream

The last product to custom-design is the final protectant. Most estheticians think of this as the day cream. If the facial is given late at night, and the client wants to be able to go home and go straight to bed, it would make sense to create a night cream.

For the example of Ms. Jones' facial, the formulation for her final finishing treatment:

Mix ½ oz. sesame, 5 drops jasmine, and 5 drops rose. Blend together and lightly massage all over face and neck.

Scheduling Follow-up Appointments

As the client goes up to the front desk to pay the bill, you or the receptionist should ask the client when to book their next facial. Try to make sure that the questions are not presented in a "yes or no" format. Human nature makes most people respond with a "no" response before a "yes." Once you and your entire staff change the way you present your questions, you will be thrilled with how many more people immediately book their appointments. Try something like this:

> "Ms. Jones what would be a convenient time to book your next facial? Your (facialist's name) notes on your card that she/he recommends that extractions should be completed in the next two weeks. If this time of day is good for you, there is an opening on a Thursday (a date, 2 weeks ahead) Would you like to schedule for then?"

Contrary to what some might think, this is not being too pushy. It has been proven that most clients will not commit to another appointment if they do not want one. This approach simply makes it easier to keep the appointments flowing. Anything can come up in the client's schedule that would make it necessary to change the appointment, or even cancel it altogether. However, if the client leaves the salon without scheduling another appointment, it may be months before he or she finds the time to call to do so.

Most estheticians have heard thousands of times over the years "I was meaning to make an appointment and time just flew by." When an appointment is made for the client at the end of the session, it is written on an appointment card. The client can slip it into a wallet or purse before leaving. They are now back on schedule and appreciating it too.

Skin Care Formulas: Cleansers and Tonics

This section provides the details for creating the special products needed to conduct an aromatherapy facial. Since skin care is so complex and has so many different areas of treatments, separate sections are offered for the most popular treatments and the most often-used products.

Aromatherapy Cleansing Formulas

Formula #1—Light-weight makeup remover: Designed for clients with sensitive eyes and/or for water-based mascara users. Use one sterile 6 oz. glass container with cap. Pour in 3 oz. aloe vera gel, 1 oz. chinese tea, and 1 drop lemon juice mixed in with 2 oz. of purified water that has been pre-mixed with 1 tablespoon of Ivory Snow powdered detergent. Put the cap on the bottle and shake to blend. Keep refrigerated to keep it fresh. (This formula will last for approximately four weeks, if refrigerated.)

Formula #2—Heavy-weight makeup remover: Designed for thick makeup users, especially for waterproof mascara users. Use one sterile 6 oz. glass container with cap. Pour in 1 oz. aloe vera gel, 1 oz. Chinese Tea, 1 oz. allantoin, 2 drops neroli, 2 drops rose, and 3 oz. of purified water that has been pre-mixed with 3 tablespoons of Ivory Snow powdered detergent. Put the cap on the bottle and shake to blend. Keep refrigerated to keep it fresh.

Formula #3—All cleansers: Begin with a base. It is recommended that each day you set up a 16 oz. bottle of this base, to be poured later into 2 oz. containers to be used for each client. If on an average day the esthetician performs more than eight facials, then two bottles should be made at the beginning of each day. It is *NOT* recommended that the esthetician try to make several batches ahead of time. Freshness should not be compromised for convenience of time. Making two bottles the evening before, and storing them in a refrigerator, should be as far in advance as you go.

Start with 8 oz. of purified water. You can boil tap water and pour it into a 16 oz. sterilized glass container. A simpler way would be to purchase a distilled bottle of water and pour 8 oz. into a sterile glass bottle. While slowly and gently stirring, add: 1 oz. of either Ivory Snow powdered detergent or Purex powdered detergent into the water. **Stir gently so as not to create bubbles.** This may clump up or appear lumpy. This is perfectly ok and will not affect the effect of the cleanser. Once you add the other ingredients and warm it up while mixing, the formula will blend smoothly. THIS IS NOW THE BASE FOR ALL THE CLEANSER FORMULATIONS.

CAUTION

Special care must be practiced when using specific oils.

Remember: Rosemary, sage, eucalyptus, hyssop, fennel, and tagetes (among others) are **very dangerous** to pregnant women.

Eucalyptus and lemongrass **cannot** be used on young children.

Bergamot is **very dangerous** to any client with photosensitivity.

> **NOTE**
>
> All the formulas will work for the specific skin type. The preference becomes most apparent in the natural fragrances that each create. The most noticeable reactions to each recipe, based on actual reactions, are given. You must experiment to find what will work best for your clients.

Formula #4—All Purpose Skin Care Cleanser: Use a baby bottle warmer. Place the sterile glass beaker inside and add: 8 drops cider vinegar, 6 drops almond, 6 drops chamomile, and 6 drops lemongrass. Stir until mixed. Then slowly add the 2 oz. of the base (Formula #3).

This formula will not be sudsy. It will have a smooth sensation. The skin will feel squeaky clean. Perfect for the client who is looking for a natural cleanser.

Formula #5—Acne Skin Cleaner: Use the baby bottle warmer. Place the sterile glass beaker inside and add: 2 drops bergamot, 4 drops lavender, 4 drops juniper, and 2 drops rosemary. Stir until mixed. Then slowly add the 2 oz. of the base (Formula #3).

This formula cleans the skin deep down. The skin can have a mild tingle to it, depending on how sensitive the skin is before the cleaning process begins.

Variation A—Formula #5: Start by adding: 8 drops palmarosa, 2 drops peppermint, and 4 drops sandalwood. Stir until mixed. Then slowly add the 2 oz. of the base (Formula #3).

For the clients who want to feel that zesty, just-washed feeling, this is for them. The skin will most often tingle for a few minutes after the cleanser has finished its job. This blend is a wonderful example of using top, middle, and base notes together.

Variation B—Formula #5: Start by adding: 2 drops clary sage, 4 drops lemon oil, and 6 drops violet leaf oil. Stir until mixed. Then slowly add the 2 oz. of the base.

This is a mild cleanser for actively acned skin. Particularly helpful for those clients who are sensitive to any tingle sensation.

Variation C—Formula #5: Start by adding: 8 drops eucalyptus, 2 drops juniper, and 2 drops patchouli. Stir until mixed. Then slowly add the 2 oz. of the base.

The eucalyptus leaves the skin feeling full of spirit. The patchouli leaves the skin feeling refreshed.

> **NOTE**
> For the esthetician with more advanced skills in aromatherapy treatments, remember the guideline to keep your formulations from becoming overpowering is to keep the mixing of oils to a maximum of 4. The second guideline is to keep the concentration to an even mix, or to have one selected oil be twice as concentrated as the others.

A partial list of the essential oils known to be effective for **acne facial skin** includes: bergamot, eucalyptus, juniper, lavender, lemon oil, palmarosa, patchouli, peppermint, petitgrain, rosemary, sandalwood, thyme, and violet leaf oil.

Formula #6—Dry Skin Cleanser: Use the baby bottle warmer. Place the sterile glass beaker inside and add: 8 drops almond oil, 4 drops avocado oil, and 4 drops grapeseed oil. Stir until mixed. Then slowly add the 2 oz. of the base (Formula #3).

The client's skin will feel clean and a lot softer. This is a mild cleanser. It is a good example of how the base oils can be effective without the use of added essential oils.

Variation A—Formula #6: Start by adding: 16 drops almond oil, 2 drops clary sage, and 2 drops lemon oil. Stir until mixed. Then slowly add the 2 oz. of the base (Formula #3).

This is great for clients who need to feel that they are not doing anything different than usual. Some clients do not want to feel that their cleaning process is noticeable, this will work for them.

Variation B—Formula #6: Start by adding: 20 drops cocoa butter and 10 drops grapeseed oil. Stir until mixed. Then slowly add the 2 oz. of the base.

For a client with very dry skin, this is perfect. It is also great for those clients who have used any kind of "cold-cream" cleanser.

Variation C—Formula #6: Start by adding: 4 drops clary sage, 4 drops jasmine and 4 drops rose. Stir until mixed. Then slowly add the 2 oz. of the base.

This formula has a light flowery fragrance. Women like this cleanser more than men.

Variation D—Formula #6: Start by adding: 12 drops palmarosa, 8 drops rosemary, and 4 drops rose. Stir until mixed. Then slowly add the 2 oz. of the base.

This also has a floral scent to it. It is light in texture, too.

Variation E—Formula #6: Start by adding: 4 drops jasmine, 4 drops rose, and 8 drops sandalwood. Stir until mixed. Then slowly add the 2 oz. of the base.

This cleanser has a woodsy fragrance and is more apt to appeal to men or anyone who enjoys the outdoors.

A partial list of the essential oils known to be effective for **dry facial skin** includes: benzoin, carrot, chamomile, geranium, hyssop, neroli, patchouli, palmarosa, rose, and sandalwood.

Formula #7—Oily Skin Cleanser: Use the baby bottle warmer. Place the sterile glass beaker inside and add: 4 drops clary sage, 8 drops geranium, and 12 drops lemon oil. Stir until mixed. Then slowly add the 2 oz. of the base (Formula #3).

This cleanser leaves the skin feeling clean and smooth, without a filmy residue.

Variation A—Formula #7: Start by adding: 4 drops frankincense, 4 drops lavender, and 8 drops ylang-ylang. Stir until mixed. Then slowly add the 2 oz. of the base (Formula #3).

This formula generally has a strong impact on the client's nose. It will either be liked a lot, or not at all. Have clients smell the frankincense BEFORE you begin to mix this one together.

Variation B—Formula #7: Start by adding: 4 drops benzoin, 4 drops carrot, and 8 drops cypress. Stir until mixed. Then slowly add the 2 oz. of the base.

Men love this formula. The fragrance is almost nonexistent. The benzoin leaves the skin ever so mildly tingly.

Variation C—Formula #7: Start by adding: 4 drops jasmine, 4 drops marjoram, and 4 drops patchouli. Stir until mixed. Then slowly add the 2 oz. of the base.

The oriental essence of this cleanser might make your clients feel like they have stepped back into time. It has a romantic aura to it. This is a popular cleanser with older clients.

A partial list of the essential oils known to be effective for **oily facial skin** includes: carrot, chamomile, clary sage, cypress, frankincense, geranium, jasmine, lavender, petitgrain, and ylang-ylang.

Formula 8—Sensitive Skin Cleanser: Use the baby bottle warmer. Place the sterile glass beaker inside and add: 4 drops carrot, 8 drops geranium, and 4 drops lemon oil. Stir until mixed. Then slowly add the 2 oz. of the base (Formula #3).

As the skin type indicates, this cleanser is light. It is not a great choice for the client who wears heavy makeup.

Variation A—Formula #8: Start by adding: 1 drop hyssop, 4 drops lavender, and 8 drops lemon oil. Stir until mixed. Then slowly add the 2 oz. of the base (Formula #3).

The client will be able to smell this cleanser, so first check out the client's reaction to hyssop. Notice that there is only one drop of hyssop used. It works better to get the makeup off, and it is not as mild as Formula #8.

Variation B—Formula #8: Start by adding: 2 drops chamomile, 4 drops jasmine and 4 drops neroli. Stir until mixed. Then slowly add the 2 oz. of the base.

This is a very gentle cleanser and will be a favorite of many clients.

Variation C—Formula #8: Start by adding: 15 drops rosewood, 2 drops patchouli and 6 drops lemon oil. Stir until mixed. Then slowly add the 2 oz. of the base.

This will have an essence that resembles a cologne. It appeals to older women more than young girls.

Variation D—Formula #8: Start by adding: 4 drops geranium, 4 drops palmarosa, and 4 drops carrot. Stir until mixed. Then slowly add the 2 oz. of the base.

Similar to Variation C, it will appeal to an older clientele.

A partial list of the essential oils known to be effective for **sensitive facial skin** includes: carrot, chamomile, geranium, hyssop, jasmine, lavender, neroli, palmarosa, patchouli, rose, rosewood, and sandalwood.

Formulas for Skin Care Tonics and Rinses

In pre-made regular products, astringents and toners are the same thing, respectively, as tonics and rinses. In aromatherapy, the products are made up of essential oils that possess the natural abilities to work on the skin as an astringent or toner. You can also mix essential oils and other plant parts to create an entire formula.

NOTE
Refrigerate all formulations when not in use.

As in the aromatherapy skin care cleanser formulations, beginners and the more advanced estheticians are provided the formulation information to use themselves.

CAUTION

When applying tonics, always cover the client's eyes, and shake each mixture thoroughly before spraying.

Acne Skin Tonic

Formula #1: Mix 3 oz. of witch hazel with 1 oz. St. Johns Wort, add 8 drops patchouli, 4 drops clary sage, and 4 drops palmarosa. Put into a sprayer bottle.

Perky is a good word to describe the reaction the skin will feel after this is used on it.

Formula #2: Start with 4 oz. of witch hazel and add 2 drops bergamot, and 5 drops thyme. Put into a sprayer bottle.

This tonic will leave the skin very tingly. Most clients will feel its kick. It will not be a negative reaction, just a strong one. CHECK WITH THE CLIENT TO MAKE SURE THAT THEY ARE NOT GOING OUT INTO THE SUN.

Formula #3—for Rosacea: Mix 3 oz. witch hazel with 1 oz. cider vinegar. Add 2 drops bergamot and 4 drops clary sage. Put into a sprayer bottle.

This formula is perfect for treating irritation of the skin. It will be mild for most people and maybe slightly perky for sensitive types.

Other Tonics

Formula #4—Dry Skin Tonic: Mix 3½ oz. Chinese Tea and ½ oz. of witch hazel. Add 4 drops chamomile, and 4 drops sandalwood. Put into a sprayer bottle.

This is a wonderful tonic for anyone with dry skin. It will leave the skin clean and have no topical reaction at all. Everyone loves this one.

Formula #5—Oily Skin Tonic: Mix 4 oz. witch hazel with 8 drops lemon oil. Add 8 drops lemon juice and 3 drops geranium. Put into a sprayer bottle.

For active clients with oily skin, this tonic is a life saver. It has a clean, fresh smell that they like, too.

Formula #6—Sensitive Skin Tonic: Mix 4 oz. Chinese Tea with 1 drop hyssop, 4 drops chamomile, and 2 drops sandalwood. Put into a sprayer bottle.

This formula is perfect as a tonic that will not leave the skin red. The only precaution that you might want to take, is checking the client's reaction to hyssop. Most love the woodsy smell of sandalwood.

Aromatherapy Masks

This section covers the concepts important to understanding the masking process, along with the various methods that are available to use the process in many different facial treatments.

There are two basic concepts of masking. One that pulls from the skin, and one that puts into the skin. Both can be part of the aromatherapy program. What surprises a lot of estheticians is that dry skin can improve with the use of certain clay packs. Dry skin has many dead cells that need to be removed. The pulling power of clay can do this very evenly. With aromatherapy, the esthetician has total control over the intensity of the clay, as well as the ability to customize the formula by adding other ingredients to revitalize the dry skin at the same time.

The key ingredient for all masks that pull out of the skin, is some kind of biological clay. The most commonly used is kaolin and/or soft brown clay. Some comes from the mud found in the sea. The clay can be found all over the world. It comes in many different colors, red, brown, white, yellow, green and black. Although clay has the strength and power to work as treatment by itself, adding essential oils to the clay make it more effective, and more specialized, for each client.

As previously mentioned, aromatherapy gives the masks the ability to be blended so that they add elements to the surface of the skin. The three key elements are water, nutrients/vitamins, and hormones. The first is easier to see outright. The latter two are found in essential oils. These masks are more often used on dry, mature skin. Any client, regardless of the skin type, can find these helpful if they are using Retin-A, have had any form of cosmetic surgery, or are experiencing direct skin trauma, such as a sunburn. These masks add moisture to the surface so quickly, in fact, that the texture will change after just one treatment. (Formulations for these masks are detailed in Chapter 8.)

In dealing with clay based masks the biggest mistake estheticians make, is to overdry the masks they use on their oily-skin clients. Remember that the brain will register the loss of water from the skin and begin to produce more oil. This oil will not show up on faces until 48 hours after the treatment. Therefore, they will be away from you when it happens, and the client won't make the connection to the overdrying of the mask. In addition, they remember how dry the mask felt when they were in the facial room, and will repeat the exact same process with their home-care regimen during the masking phase.

"Shower Power" Home Care

This author has created a program for her personal clients, which she calls her "Shower Power." When a client decides to go through their personal skin-care regimen, there is just one place where they will get the best results. There is only one place that will allow the proper messages to be sent to the brain . . . their shower. Understanding why it works will help you share it with your own clients and friends. Everyone's face has fine vellum hair follicles that act as sensors for many different stimuli. The amount of water in the surface of the skin is tracked by these vellum hair follicles. The brain will not easily release oil out of the pores, if it determines that this oil will be needed later for lack of hydration.

During a facial treatment, the esthetician will use a steamer. The fine mist lays on the vellum and sends a temporary message through that there is indeed enough water, and so extracting the oil from the pores is easy. For the client's homecare regimen, it is ONLY WHEN THEY ARE IN A SHOWER, that the vellum are given the same message. Thus this author has created the "SHOWER POWER" programs to utilize the effects of the moisture that hangs in the air while in the shower. The client is instructed to apply their mask while in the shower, and remove it at the END OF THE SHOWER. No need to time it other than that. Some people take long showers and others short ones. Either will work just fine. The quality of time and consistency will make a bigger impact than trying to find 20–30 minutes every two or three weeks. This program can be done once or twice a week with better results taking the excess oil, skin and toxins off of the skin.

Chapter 8

Specific Skin Conditions and Formulas

Every working cosmetologist and esthetician finds themselves having to deal with many different skin conditions and problems. This text provides detailed holistic explanations for the reasons why so many of these conditions and problems exist. The information is designed to inform and enlighten the reader on the way the body is understood from the viewpoint of a holistic practitioner. For each condition, an appropriate aromatherapy treatment and formula is also explained.

NOTE

For the esthetician with more advanced skills in aromatherapy treatments, remember the guideline to keep your formulations from becoming overpowering is to keep the mixing of oils to a maximum of four. The second guideline is to keep the concentration to an even mix or to have one selected oil be twice as concentrated as the others.

CAUTION

Special care must be practiced when using specific oils.

Remember: Rosemary, sage, eucalyptus, hyssop, fennel, and tagetes (among others) are **very dangerous** to pregnant women.

Eucalyptus and lemongrass **cannot** be used on young children.

Bergamot is **very dangerous** to any client with photo-sensitivity.

Dry, Flaky Skin

The most misunderstood condition is that of dry, flaky skin. It is the one condition that keeps the annual sales of moisturizers in the billions of dollars. Cosmetic manufacturers are counting on a misconception that has been maintaining itself for a very long time (with the help of advertisers). Although the truth is not overly popular, it must be told: If clients would control their diet in specific ways, they would never have dry flaky skin!

It all starts with the physical makeup of the body. The human body and the planet are both comprised of 70% water concentration. Both are capable of experiencing droughts. The skin has no way of creating any water within itself. External sources are required. The daily balance of consumption is 64 oz. (eight 8 oz. glasses), is needed if a person just stays around the house and does nothing more than read or watch television. When you add any form of activity, going to work, shopping, taking care of children etc., the amount of water needed for total hydration balance increases by 1 oz. an hour. That amount increases if the activity causes the body to break out into a sweat. For example, for one hour of a gym workout, the average fluid loss is 8 oz. per hour for women and 12–14 oz. for men.

Remember the brain's number one rule: "Above all else, keep this body alive." Since water is needed in every single molecule of the body in order for it to stay healthy, the skin is not given a high priority in the brain's water distribution hierarchy. This is why everyone has to keep drinking water.

Also cutting down on salt, alcoholic beverages and all caffeinated drinks like coffee, tea, and soft drinks will help a client's body stay water-rich. Juices and soups will add water into our diets, but these two have to be digested first before the water content is available. Water is the only substance that does not break down in the stomach. Proof is found in intravenous glucose feedings in hospitals. Patients are given sugar water directly into their veins.

The Hard Part: Getting on a "Water Schedule"

Sometimes encouraging words and caveats aren't enough. The following describes the author's method of getting her clients on a water-drinking schedule.

First, instruct your clients to purchase the most attractive glass they can afford. This will play a major role to getting them started. Eyes will be drawn to a gorgeous, cut crystal goblet or household glass, versus a styrofoam cup!

Second, instruct that the water be fresh, slightly chilled, not too cold, with a slice of fresh lemon, lime or orange peel to add flavor and scent to the water. Even bottled water will be more enjoyable with a rind sliver added.

Third, let yoiur clients know that the water schedule is the most important part to making water a permanent part of their lives. The most often asked question is "Will I find myself running to the bathroom all day if I do this?" And the answer is no, if it is followed properly.

The client is told to drink one 8 oz. glass of water the first and second day. The client can take all day to drink it. Although if done that slowly it will make the rest of the program more difficult to complete. Then two glasses for two more days. Three glasses for three days. Four glasses for four days. Five glasses for five days. At this intake level, the client's tongue will become parched without the daily water consumption. This makes it easier to continue when the body helps remind them. Then six glasses for six days. Seven glasses for seven days and finally eight glasses for eight days and all following days. Your client is now on the way to staying healthier and slimmer; with shinier hair, stronger nails, and smooth, soft, and moist skin!

Nature's Alternative Moisture

Since the body needs so much water, and the skin does not always get its fair share, nature has provided the skin with an alternative to keep moist. The **sebaceous glands** play a key role in keeping the skin smooth and soft. The size of the oil glands are set at birth. We can never change them. The **pore** is the opening at end of the long follicular channel connected directly to the gland. The larger the gland, the wider the channel, which means the pore will be wider. Think of it like a straw connected to the end of a pump. The larger the pump, the wider the straw would have to be to let the oil out.

> If you learn only one thing from this book, please let it be that **pores do not open and close** like your fist can. Pore size is not determined by what products you use or do not use! The activity level of the oil gland has a direct effect on the amount of expansion of the follicular channel, and thus, the width of the pore up until the age of 50. Once a person reaches 50 years of age, the weakening of all collagen and elastin fibers will have a direct effect on the ap-

pearance of the pores. As the skin's netting weakens, a noticeable difference in the appearance of the pores is created.

Regardless of what the jar, tube or bottle says: NO products will change the actual size of the pore. What can happen is that the product can cause minor edemas (swelling) around the pore opening. While the swelling condition is present, the pore opening will appear smaller. Once the swelling subsides, the appearance of the pore returns to its original size. The pore itself never changed.

There are lifestyle choices that will cause the skin to be water deficient. Two situations qualify for the number one reason: smoking and drinking alcoholic beverages. Both get into the blood stream and cause a great imbalance of water. Remember, you cannot get your client to stop these two habits unless they want too! Aromatherapy will help temporarily rid the skin of these toxins.

Remember that the seasons will have a direct effect on the water level of each of your client's skin. Aromatherapy offers you the flexibility to customize as the seasons change. In addition, the clients who do a lot of traveling are faced with many climatic changes. They will love being able to come to you to "fix" all that traveling takes out of their skin. Aromatherapy aids in developing client retention, based on their being dependent on you for the treatment "formula."

Aromatherapy Formulas for DRY SKIN

Formula #1: Start with 1 oz. avocado oil and add: 4 drops patchouli, 4 drops rose and 4 drops neroli. Blend together, then use deep massage techniques to penetrate it into the skin.

"Smooth" and "sleek" are adjectives that describe this formula's reaction to the skin. The floral bouquet fragrance is very pleasant.

Formula #2: Start with 1 oz.wheatgerm oil and add: 10 drops lavender, 1 drop hyssop and 5 drops rosemary. Blend together, then use deep massage techniques to penetrate it into the skin.

Milder in fragrance, this formula also leaves the skin smooth.

Formula #3: Start with 1 oz. apricot oil and add: 6 drops sandalwood, 3 drops rose, and 3 drops neroli. Blend together, then use deep massage techniques to penetrate it into the skin.

The woodsy fragrance will appeal to the outdoors advocate.

Formula #4: Start with 1 oz. olive oil and add: 5 drops carrot, 5 drops chamomile, and 5 drops geranium. Blend together, then use deep massage techniques to penetrate it into the skin.

If leaving the skin satiny without a lingering smell is what you want, then this will work well.

A partial list of the essential oils known to be effective for **dry facial skin** includes: benzoin, carrot, chamomile, geranium, hyssop, neroli, patchouli, palmarosa, rose, rosemary, and sandalwood.

Excessively Oily Skin and Texture

The size of the oil glands are set at birth. Nothing can change this. The oil glands begin to activate around the age of 8 and get into full production capability around puberty. This varies by individual, but the average age of onset is between 11 and 13. Just like the varing degrees of height, there are many different degrees of glandular size. The larger the glands, the higher the volume capability of oil production. No one can actually look "into the skin" to determine what size glands are there. There are two ways to help determine what size oil wells are under the skin.

The first determinant is heredity. If one of the parents has large oil glands, the child has a greater than 50% chance to have large glands. If both parents have large oil glands, then their offspring have a 100% chance of having large oil glands.

The second determinant is the size of the pores. The pore size is connected to the size of the oil glands. The pores are the ends of the follicular channels that are directly connected to the oil glands. Large pore openings register large oil glands. Small pores register small ones.

Here is one way to explain oil production levels as it relates to the size of the sebaceous glands: Imagine in one hand you have an 8 oz. glass and in the other, a 4 oz. juice glass. If both were filled to the very top and spilled over, the puddle from the large glass would be more to clean up.

Size is not the only factor in how active the glands will be. The percentage of production is the other part of the equation. Using the glasses as the example, if both are only half-full of water, and you are very thirsty, the 4 oz. glass will be less helpful to you because there will be so much less water to drink.

Contributing Factors to Oil Production

Whether the glands are producing at 100% or at less than full capacity is largely influenced by age. Oil production reduces around 35 years of age. The reduction is slow at first, and therefore not always noticed. The decrease follows a five-year time line.

The skin's oil pattern follows like this: at the age of 20, a freshly washed face would show signs of oil production in less than one hour. At 30, it would take the skin to show oil in two hours. At 35, 3–4 hours, at 40, 4–6 hours, at 45, 6–8 hours. The exact level of decrease has never been scientifically measured.

There are other factors controlling the skin's degree of oil production. The first deals with the body's need for moisture. There is a huge difference between being water dehydrated and oil deficient. The need for water has a direct effect on the production level of the sebaceous gland. If the client makes a change in the intake of fluids, particularly water, it will have an impact in reducing the glandular secretion level. (Refer back to the water drinking program set out in the previous section.)

Oily skin has a different texture than dry skin. With this condition, the client has potentially more control over the skin's ability to improve its overall appearance and texture. Aromatherapy treatments offer the client the opportunity to reduce the "orange peel" look of oily skin. When the skin has too much oil coming to the surface, the individual pores swell and an "orange peel" appearance takes over. It is most often prominent in the area around the nose and cheek. Essential oils improve the feel of the skin by degreasing the surface and returning the outer layer to a smoother texture. Whether brought about by lifestyle choices or heredity, aromatherapy offers solutions for improvement.

There are also environmental factors to consider. Smoking has a direct impact on the production level of the glands. Therefore, a child of parents with very oily skin should reconsider starting the habit. In addition to basic health reasons, anyone who is interested in having a clear complexion should not smoke. Although clinical studies are not complete as of the printing of this book, it may be proven that secondhand smoke has a direct, negative impact on the skin and oil productivity.[1]

Another impact on the sebaceous glandular activity is the level of alcohol in the bloodstream. Particularly important are the patterns of consumption where larger amounts of alcohol are ingested over a short period of time, but done repeatedly. For example: clients who drink consistently on the weekends, as part of their social activity. Clients in their twenties may fall into this pattern. In the beginning of the week, their skin has to deal with the dehydration the alcohol creates internally, which forces the glands to work extra hard, pushing higher volumes of oil to the surface. The weekend comes along again, and the pattern repeats itself. These clients will come to the esthetician complaining of how oily their skin is all the time.

Hormones are another part of the reasons for oily skin textures. For female clients, with heavy periods, and/or premenstrual syndrome, the sebaceous glands react sharply to when the other hormone levels rise. There are strong internal connections throughout the eccrine system. The sebaceous glands are part of the system, along with the sudiferous, thyroid, adrenal, lymphatic, hyperthymus, ovaries (in women), and prostate (in men). Every time there is a surge in the release inside of the ovaries, the activity level in the sebaceous glands rise too. For the average woman under 40, it is roughly every 28 days. For men it is every 3 days. Similarly, the whole system reacts to other emotional stimuli. If a client was driving on a freeway and an unexpected event occured, like being cut off without any warning, their heart would feel like it got a jolt, because their adrenal glands would release adrenaline into the bloodstream. At that same moment, the sebaceous glands would be triggered too. In less than 48 hours, their face would be showing the effects of that oil release.

Aromatherapy and Brain Waves

One of the marvelous effects of aromatherapy is its ability to be a stress reducer. Aromatherapy applications can send signals of relaxation to the brain. Since stress can have a direct impact on the oil level of the skin, aromatherapy treatments will control the immediate coatings on the surface of the skin, and help the client deal with stress level too.

The effects of essential oils on brain waves patterns are being studied by researchers. Under careful observations, patients have inhaled certain oil's natural aromas. Basil, rosemary, and peppermint are just three essential oils known for their ability to stimulate clarity of thought and produce more beta brain waves. These waves indicate increased alertness. Jasmine and neroli are two essential oils that act as antidepressants by their increase of the production of alpha, delta, and theta waves.[2]

Self-esteem is an integral part of mental health. Aromatherapy can add to a person's feeling of being in control with the increase of certain brain waves. During a facial, the esthetician can work with essential oils to bring about a physical and psychological response.

Having this power at your fingertips is just one of the many reasons aromatherapy is growing in popularity among the professionals in salons seeking to stay current with the best services available.

Being able to offer immediate results to your clients is a real strong reason aromatherapy will work for you. Using aromatherapy treatments as part of your program to treat oily skin texture problems raises your confidence in your results. Your clients sense your level of confidence in your work.

Aromatherapy Formulations for Oily Skin

Formula #1: Use the baby bottle warmer. Place the sterile glass beaker inside and start with 1 oz. ginseng tea and add: 4 drops clary sage, 8 drops geranium, and 12 drops lemon oil. Stir until mixed. Then slowly massage into the face, neck and décolleté area.

This is a very lightweight formula, and the client will like the fresh feeling it leaves.

Formula #2: Start with 1 oz. aloe vera juice and add: 4 drops frankincense, 4 drops lavender, and 8 drops ylang-ylang. Stir until mixed. Then slowly massage into the face, neck and décolleté area.

Check the client's reaction to frankincense first. This will have an exotic sensation on/in the nose. The clients either are mystified by it or repelled by it.

Formula #3: Start with 1 oz. ginseng tea and add: 4 drops benzoin, 4 drops carrot, and 8 drops cypress. Stir until mixed. Then slowly massage into the face, neck and décolleté area.

This is a very lightweight formula and a real winner with men.

Formula #4: Start with 1 oz. of ginger root juice and add: 4 drops jasmine, 4 drops marjoram, and 4 drops patchouli. Stir until mixed. Then, slowly massage into the face, neck and décolleté area.

The lightweight action of this oil appeals to younger clientele. The oriental fragrance is a winner with a lot of people.

A partial list of the essential oils known to be effective for **oily facial skin** includes: benzoin, carrot, chamomile, clary sage, cypress, frankincense, geranium, jasmine, lavender, palmarosa, patchouli, petitgrain, and ylang-ylang.

Aromatherapy Mask Formulas for Purging Oily Skin

The clays used in aromatherapy masks can be found all over the world. The clay comes in many different colors: red, brown, white, yellow, green and black. Although clay has the strength and power to work as a treatment by itself, adding essential oils to it makes it more effective. Essential oils also make each clay mask more specialized for each client.

Each mask must have a base. This base is what is used with all the various other ingredients to make up the final products. The formulas are for one singular application.

Clay Mask Base Formula

Begin by using the baby bottle warmer. Place the sterile glass beaker inside and start with 1 heaping tablespoon of corn starch, 2 tsp. of brewer's yeast and add 3 tbsp. of kaolin clay (white clay). Stir all three powders, blending evenly. This is the base for all of the "pulling" mask formulations.

While stirring, slowly add 1 oz. of purified water. Stir thoroughly to make the paste the consistency of smooth peanut butter. Once blended, slowly add: 1 oz. more of the purified water, if you are only going to coat the face. If you are including the neck, add one more ounce of water, stirring slowly as you add it. These four ingredients become the base.

NOTE

You may use distilled, bottled water. Spring water will also work well. Try to stay away from using tap water or well water. Both will have added deposits that will not necessarily be helpful to your treatment.

Formula #1: Start with the base. Add: 3 drops eucalyptus, 1 drop peppermint, and 1 drop thyme. Blend well. Apply over the face with a fan brush. Leave on the skin for 5–7 minutes. Remove with a warm towel. (Pre-heat towels in a crockery cooking pot. Then they will be ready anytime.) Spray the skin with an oily skin tonic.

This mask's effectiveness is in the skin's strong reaction to it. The client will feel it doing its work soon after it touches the skin. This formula is a bit unusual in that it uses three powerful essential oils—all top notes—but uses only small amounts of each.

Formula #2: Start with the base. Add: 1 drop bergamot, 3 drops juniper, and 3 drops lemon oil. Follow the same application technique as mentioned above in Formula #1.

Also a great mask, but there will not be as strong sensations to its application. Notice that only one drop of bergamot is used. Still make sure the client is NOT going out in the sun.

Formula #3: Start with the base. Add: 5 drops petitgrain, 5 drops sandalwood, and 5 drops patchouli. Follow the same application technique as mentioned in Formula #1.

The woodsy fragrance of this mask will be perfect for all your physically active clients. They will love having this on their face. Using two base note oils with an equal amount of a top note oil rounds out this formulation.

Formula #4: Start with the base: Add 8 drops lavender, 8 drops juniper, and 8 drops thyme. Follow the same application technique as mentioned above in Formula #1.

The thyme will tingle but not by much. It is not advisable to use this much thyme if the formula was going to penetrate into the skin. As a mask it stays on top of the skin, so should not be a problem. The mask will do a nice job of cleaning, without a lot of fanfare.

A partial list of the essential oils known to be effective for **"pulling" masks for oily facial skin** includes: bergamot, eucalyptus, juniper, lavender, lemon oil, palmarosa, patchouli, peppermint, petitgrain, rosemary, sandalwood, thyme, and violet.

Mature, Lined Skin

Billions of dollars are spent each year in attempts to temper the ravages of time against the face and body. As of the writing of this book, there are no true "miracle cures." But there have been many breakthroughs that, ironically, have their roots in aromatherapy.

In the eighties, liposomes were introduced into the cosmetic industry as vehicles for deeper penetration of products into the skin. The liposome would be able to take an animal fat protein and force it deeper into the stratum corneum layer of the epidermal tissue. Various different collagen sources were introduced the same way.

Aromatherapy uses plant life to do the same thing. And it is because all plant life has an oxygen connection, even after it has been removed from the ground, that makes the essential oil system so unique and effective. Every molecule of our body needs oxygen. Tapping into the essential oils' sources makes the entry into our bodies so easy. You must have a thorough understanding of how the skin keeps its shape to better understand how the esthetician helps to maintain it.

Inside the second layer of skin, the dermis, is where **collagen** and **elastin** fibers are produced. You can think of these two parts as close sisters that do everything together. Each has their own characteristics, but they work well together to make up the fibrous network of the skin. Think of the collagen fibers as asparagus stalks and the elastin fibers as the rubber bands that keep the stalks together. As they grow old, the stalks get dry, brittle, and snap into smaller disconnected pieces, and the rubber band dries out, losing its ability to be flexible and hold the stalks in place.

Through medical technology, collagen injections have been created and used to boost the skin's collagen levels. The use of collagen injections falls into the medical community's responsibility and therefore will not be covered in any further detail. In regard to aromatherapy, the use of essential oils offers nutrients and proteins that work to restore these important tissue fibers. Essential oils can prevent toxins from collecting in the skin by expediting the elimination process completed through the lymphatic system. They improve the circulation, which aids oxygenation and energizes the dermis by the rate the nutrients are fed into it, through the absorption of the essential oils when massaged into the skin. In some cases the change in the person's texture is so dramatic, it appears as if the client has had a facelift.

Aromatherapy offers painless, safe solutions for improved elasticity that do not require the client to have surgery. This is a very strong reason to offer it as part of your services.

As of this writing, the newest breakthrough has been in alpha hydroxyacids, otherwise known as AHAs. There are several different kinds: from citric acids, which come from oranges, lemons and limes; to tartaric acid from grapes; lactic acid from sour milk; to glycolic acid, which comes from sugar cane or sugar beets.

It is the last AHA, the glycolic acid, of which the most hoopla has been made. It is the smallest molecule of the lot and therefore gets furthest into the skin's system to aid the cellular turnover of the tissue. (Remember that as the skin ages, it takes longer for the cells to climb to the surface. And the amount of stronger, healthier cells diminish with time, too.) It is the essential oil elements inside of the glycolic acid that make it work so well and so fast. Technology has provided the esthetician with a powerful tool. Glycolic acids have the power of the essential oils' full strength and the intensity of the solutions' strength.

Currently, the esthetician is allowed to use up to 40% glycolic acid strength without a doctor being on the premises. With a physician's assistance, i.e. working in a medical clinic, the solution can be as powerful as 70%. The esthetician can use the glycolic acid as a treatment alone, or incorporate it with a complete aromatherapy facial.

The glycolic acid peels the skin, several layers at a time. The internal mechanisms of the dermis registers the removal of the cells and speeds up production to create new ones. This cellular activity is what creates the new appearance of the face. And it is this improvement that has caused so much excitement in the cosmetic industry. For the first time, estheticians have been given such a strong, effective tool that plays a direct role in the improvement of the client's aging appearance.

As yet, there has been no greater technological breakthrough as important as AHA's. It is important to note that the use of grapes and milk for skin rejuvenation has been recorded in history as far back as Cleopatra. Egyptian mummies have been tested to show that essential oils were used to preserve the skin. As reminded by the cliche: "Everything old is new again," aromatherapy has been brought to the forefront as the new rage for antiaging. It still works, but it is far from new.

Aromatherapy is not effective on the shortening of a flabby muscle that has atrophied over time. Only a plastic surgeon can go in and cut and re-sew the muscles back together. Essential oils do add oxygen into the muscle tissue, making them healthier. Essential oils aid in muscle tone through the reduction of toxins that otherwise would collect in the tissue.

The seasons, too, will have direct effects on the appearance of mature, lined skin. The water level of each of your client's skin is directly affected by the weather. It is particularly hardest on the skin of an older person. Aromatherapy offers you the flexibility to customize formulas as the seasons change.

Aromatherapy Formulas for Mature, Lined Skin

Formula #1: Use the baby bottle warmer. Place the sterile glass beaker inside and start with 1 oz. hazelnut oil and add: 6 drops clary sage, 12 drops geranium, and 12 drops lemon oil. Stir until mixed. Then slowly massage into the face, neck and décolleté area.

The use of lemon oil on the mature skin will have a wonderful brightening effect. The skin will look healthier.

Formula #2: Start with 1 oz. almond oil and add: 4 drops frankincense, 4 drops lavender, and 8 drops yarrow. Stir until mixed. Then slowly massage into the face, neck and décolleté area.

This formula is either a great big hit or miss with your older client.

Formula #3: Start with 1 oz. apricot oil and add: 1 drop hyssop, 4 drops rose, and 8 drops sandalwood. Stir until mixed. Then slowly massage into the face, neck and décolleté area.

The same falls true for this formula as it does with Formula #2. That's the beauty of aromatherapy, you have so many choices to create.

Formula #4: Start with 1 oz. hazelnut oil and add: 4 drops evening primrose, 1 drop fennel, and 4 drops patchouli. Stir until mixed. Then slowly massage into the face, neck and décolleté area.

The natural fragrance of this formula often appeals to your older male clients. Women who love to go walking or hiking will like it too. An area of confusion in aromatherapy often comes in the use of herbs that are regularly used in food recipes. Like basil, fennel is used in very tiny amounts in cooking water. It is a powerful herb that has many fine properties, but must also be used carefully.

A partial list of the essential oils known to be effective for **mature, lined facial skin** includes: borage seed, carrot, clary sage, evening primrose, fennel, frankincense, galbanum, geranium, hyssop, jojoba, lavender, lemon oil, lime, myrrh, neroli, orange, oregano, palmarosa, patchouli, rose, rosemary, rosewood, sandalwood, thyme, vervaine, violet leaf oil, and yarrow.

Many of the essential oils derived from herbs must be used in small amounts. They are very potent substances.

Aromatherapy Nourishing Masks for Mature, Lined Skin

Nourishing masks are designed NOT TO DRY. An added benefit is this one characteristic offers a busy esthetician, is having the freedom to leave the client with the mask on and do other services. Drying times for other masks are like clocks for the client, the dryness tells them when they "are done," and if you are not back in time, they feel like they have been deserted, or neglected. Since the client will not be able to know when the nourishing mask is ready to be removed, the esthetician is free to elongate the processing time.

Using nourishing masks can also work in favor of the esthetician in the opposite manner. The esthetician can shorten the time the mask is on the face, and the client will not know or be suspicious. Situations where this would be beneficial are when you are running behind and want to "catch up," or when the client is running late getting into the salon, potentially ruining the rest of your schedule. You can shorten the masking process, thus being ready for the next client. It is recommended that you NOT mention that you are shortening the masking time. At the end of the facial, should the client say something about getting out at the regularly scheduled time, politely say "Why yes, I wanted to keep us on track, so I made you a very special mask today." Then leave it at that.

Creating the Base for Non-Drying Gel Masks

The masks are individually formulated for single applications. Unlike the clay base, this base does not have to be the same for all of the formulations. There is, however, one ingredient that you can always count on: aloe vera gel, it is ready to use, instantly.

The following will need distilled water to be added to them, even before the other essential oils are added: ginger root, tapioca starch powder, seaweed, carrageenan, slippery elm bark powder.

You will be creating 2 oz. of the finished base for the purpose of this masking process. For any of the above-mentioned powders, slowly mix one ounce of powder to 3 oz. of distilled purified water. When mixed together, it bulks up and makes the final paste gel.

It is important to start with the powder in the beaker *first.* Slowly add the water as you continually stir the mixture. It will take some practice to get comfortable in your blending technique. And in the beginning your mask may appear lumpy. Placing it into a baby bottle warmer will assist you, however, let it cool down before you use it on the client's face. You should apply a clay mask cool, or slightly warmed, but use a gel mask cold.

These bases are designed for all the above mentioned reasons. All of these bases are used for adding water, and any nutrients, vitamins, and/or hormones. Again, the easiest base is 3 oz. of straight aloe vera gel and mixing the essential oils into it.

Aromatherapy Nourishing Masking Formulas for Mature, Lined Skin

Formula #1—Gel mask for adding moisture and reducing bacteria from the skin: Start with 2 oz. aloe vera gel and add: 10 drops patchouli, 10 drops geranium, and 5 drops ylang-ylang. Blend together and spread over the face and neck with a fan brush. Cover the face with one sheet of sterile gauze. Let set on the face for 8 minutes. Begin the removal by rolling the gauze off of the face, starting at the forehead and rolling downward towards the chin. If there is any residue left on the face, massage it into the skin. There is no need for rinsing the skin. These kind of masks are the only ones that do not need rinsing.

Formula #2—Gel mask for adding moisture, particularly for wrinkled skin: Start with 2 oz. of aloe vera gel and add: 5 drops yarrow, 5 drops sandalwood, 5 drops rose and 12 drops chamomile. Blend and follow the exact instructions as in Formula #1 above.

Formula #3—Gel mask for adding moisture and for cellular rejuvenation: Start with 2 oz. aloe vera gel and add: 15 drops rosemary, 4 drops clary sage and 4 drops lavender. Blend and follow the exact instructions as in Formula #1 above.

This is a very powerful mask. One of the more challenging goals for an esthetician is to restore vitality to aging skin. Pay close attention to the client's skin as the mask is on. You would NOT use this much rosemary in any formulation that would be massaged into the skin. As a mask, it is ok.

Formula #4—Gel mask for adding moisture for sensitive skin: Start with 2 oz. aloe vera gel and add: 8 drops carrot, 8 drops neroli, and 8 drops frankincense. Blend and follow the exact instructions as in Formula #1 above.

Aromatherapy Clay Masks for Mature, Lined Skin

One misunderstanding is that clay masks be just for oily skin. This is a very wrong assumption. With the use of aromatherapy, the esthetician can custom create the perfect clay mask for *any* type of skin. The clay described in Chapter 7 and earlier in this chapter is the same clay used for these masks.

Refer to the instructions for creating "Clay Mask Base Formula," page 117, to prepare the base for the following formulas.

One type of mask for mature, lined skin is the kind that revitalizes the moisture level.

Aromatherapy Clay Masking Formulas for Mature, Lined Skin

Formula #1: Start with the base. While stirring, add: ½ oz. of hazelnut and then 3 drops rosemary, 5 drops carrot, and 1 drop hyssop. Blend well. Apply over the face with a fan brush. Leave on the skin for 5–7 minutes. Remove with a warm towel. (Pre-heat towels in a crockery cooking pot. Then they are ready anytime.) Spray the skin with a dry skin tonic.

This mask works well on any dry skin that needs to be revitalized.

Formula #2: Start with the base. While stirring, add: ½ oz. almond oil and then 10 drops chamomile, 4 drops geranium, and 4 drops neroli. Blend well. Follow the application technique set out in Formula #1.

This formula has a broader appeal to older clientele, based on the popularity of geraniums.

Formula #3: Start with the base. While stirring, add: ½ oz. jojoba oil and then 8 drops patchouli, 4 drops sandalwood, and 2 drops benzoin. Blend well. Follow the application information in Formula #1.

This formula's woodsy aroma appeals to a lot of men.

Formula #4: Start with the base. While stirring, add: ½ oz. apricot oil and then 6 drops geranium, 2 drops rosemary, 6 drops palmarosa, and 1 drop hyssop. Blend well. Follow the application information in Formula #1.

Like others, it works great if the client's nose says YES. As always care is needed with hyssop and rosemary. The reason they are used in these formulas is because they work. It not necessary to avoid oils just because they need more care in using them. It just takes practice and common sense to develop the knowledge of how much, and when, to use the formulations.

A partial list of the essential oils known to be effective for **clay masks for dry facial skin** includes: benzoin, carrot, chamomile, geranium, hyssop, neroli, patchouli, palmarosa, rose, rosemary, and sandalwood.

Sun-damaged Skin

The sun plays an important part in the lives of all living things on the planet. Medical studies have proven that we cannot live healthy lives without some exposure and connection to the sun. Psychiatrists have proven that there is a medical condition that occurs in the brain upon prolonged absence of sun exposure, causing severe depression and dementia. So with all the medical proof of the need to be exposed to sunlight, why, of late, is it so forbidden? The answer is fairly complicated.

The sun's rays fall into three categories: ultraviolet A, ultraviolet B, and newly researched ultraviolet C. They are referred to as UV-A, UV-B and UV-C. Twenty years ago, it was thought that only the UV-B rays were the damaging kind. In fact, they were tagged as the "burning rays." However, now in the 1990s, research has uncovered that all ultraviolet rays cause some form of damage to the skin, hair, and nails, if exposure is too long during the time of day the distribution power of the sun's heat is the strongest. With the production of sunscreens, the skin can now be safely protected while the client enjoys the outdoors. One fact that is always going to be true is that sun damage stays with you for a lifetime. Most people can get a terrible sunburn at age 16, and it will heal. What they do not realize is that decades later it shows up on the aged skin. A sunburn leaves an invisible imprint in the skin. You may not see it for years, but it is still there.

An esthetician now faces clients who have sworn off exposure to the sun, now that its damaging capabilities are so well documented. Their skin will still show all the imprints of past sunburns. It is the esthetician's challenge to attempt to help relieve their client of the signs of the damage. Aromatherapy can come to their aid in a big way. If the sun damage is from years past, the tissue damage is very deep. All three UV rays have the power to penetrate all layers of the epidermal tissue. The same is true if the sunburn is new. Aromatherapy, because of it's regenerative ability, is more effective on fresh sun damage.

Essential oils are capable of penetrating all the layers of the epidermal tissue, too. Therefore, if an esthetician sees a client immediately after overexposure to the sun, they can get a head start at reducing the damage the sun will have initiated against the skin. On older sunburns or sun damage, the essential oils offer assistance to the stratum germinatum cells in regenerating.

Aromatherapy Formulas for Sun-damaged Skin

The following four formulas are for **long-term** damage:

Formula #1: Use the baby bottle warmer. Place the sterile glass beaker inside and start with 1 oz. almond oil and add: 6 drops carrot, 6 drops geranium, and 6 drops lemon oil. Stir until mixed. Then slowly massage into the face, neck and décolleté area.

This leaves the skin refreshed and the color of the skin looking terrific.

Formula #2: Start with 1 oz. sesame oil and add: 4 drops chamomile, 4 drops lavender, and 8 drops violet leaf oil. Stir until mixed. Then slowly massage into the face, neck and décolleté area.

This formula has a floral residue effect. The oils leave the skin feeling satiny.

Formula #3: Start with 1 oz. evening primrose oil and add: 12 drops neroli, 12 drops rose, and 2 drops fennel. Stir until mixed. Then slowly massage into the face, neck and décolleté area.

The power of neroli makes the skin tissue come alive. The fennel offers a romantic aura.

Formula #4: Start with 1 oz. jojoba oil and add: 2 drops peppermint, 2 drops fennel, and 2 drops galbanum. Stir until mixed. Then slowly massage into the face, neck and décolleté area.

The peppermint perks up the tired skin, the galbanum is a unique experience. Try it, they may love it.

The following formulations are for **freshly sunburned skin:**

Formula #1: Start with 1 oz. chilled aloe vera gel and add: 16 drops chamomile and 8 drops lemon oil. Stir until mixed. Dip a rolled piece of cotton that has been premoistened with ice water into the mixture. Apply formula with the cotton pad by lightly dabbing over the sunburned skin. Leave on for 5 minutes. Spray the skin with a fine mist of ice cold rosewater.

Formula #2: Start with 1 oz. chilled Chinese Tea and add: 6 drops lavender, 6 drops violet leaf oil and 2 drops carrot. Stir until mixed. Follow the same instructions as in Formula #1 above.

A partial list of the essential oils known to be effective for **sun damaged facial skin** includes: benzoin, bergamot, carrot, chamomile, cypress, fennel, galbanum, geranium, lavender, lemon oil, neroli, peppermint, rose, and violet leaf oil.

Acne

This condition generally occurs on the face, neck, back, and chest. Often, strephylococcal bacteria causes the problems of the skin. Depending on the severity of the inflammation, acne can be painful and unsightly. Hormonal fluctuation can be a main cause of acne breakouts. That is why during puberty most people experience some form of outbreak that falls into the category of Stage One Acne. Although everyone experiences the hormone rushes during puberty, it can also occur throughout one's lifetime. Thousands of women suffer monthly with premenstrual syndrome and/or heavy periods. These two situations cause tremendous hormonal fluctuations. Acne outbreaks increase during these times. This means that these women may be dealing with acne for decades.

Hormones are not the only cause for acne. Over-active sebaceous glands have a direct connection to acne. Acne is also hereditary. If both parents have had acne, then their children will have a

100% chance to have a form of acne too. Diet plays a part in acne, too. Clients should be advised to consult with a licensed nutritionist to help them create a sensible diet.

In addition, let your clients know that caffeine will have a negative effect on their skin. Smoking, salt, processed sugar, coffee, tea, alcoholic beverages and fried foods all aid in the development of impacted cells. Remember, too, that the seasons will have a direct effect on acne skin.

Acne Stages

There are four stages of acne. Minor accumulation of comedones (blackheads) on the nose and chin area are the most prominent conditions of Stage One Acne. Stages One and Two are easily dealt with in the salon's facial room. Milia (whiteheads), comedones, and minor skin plugs are signals that the client's skin is in these two stages.

Stage Three begins with low-degree infection, where pustules and pimples are flourishing in the T-zone (forehead, nose, and chin). This stage is bordering on the need of medical care. Though the advanced professional esthetician may be able to successfully extract these impactions without leaving scars and traumatized skin afterwards, it is better to leave any treatment to a doctor. Leaving the skin ripped open, torn and weakened is NOT in the best interest of the client.

Stage Four is also where the doctor must intercede if any long term treatment is needed. In this stage there are deep nodules and cysts, along with some intensely swollen pustules. The client needs to be on internal medication and their doctor's permission to have regular facials. Work with the client's doctor to determine the best treatment. This is the area that a commingling of professional talents makes working with a dermatologist very useful.

Rosacea

Rosacea is a specific form of acne that affects adults, usually in their thirties or older. The areas it affects are the nose and the cheek tissue directly next to the nose. It has two stages of progression.

During the first stage, the excessive production levels of the sebaceous glands in the sinus area causes the skin on the nose to be very greasy looking. In addition, the capillaries are irritated and constantly red and inflamed. As the inflammation becomes more intense, rosacea turns into the second stage.

In the second stage, there is the overgrowth of bacteria that form pustules that are often large and painful. The client will need internal antibiotics to get the bacteria under control. Seek permission and guidance from the client's physician before offering assistance in cleaning out the various pustules and comedones that are present. If you are not confident with your extraction skills, DO NOT ATTEMPT. Also be aware that in most rosacea patients, the scarring possibilities are so great that the patient should be on the oral medication for at least six weeks BEFORE any extractions are attempted.

Aromatherapy can offer assistance with these conditions, that traditional skin care treatments cannot. Utilizing the natural antibiotic properties of some of the essential oils will have a direct effect on the skin. Essential oils can be used to reduce the redness and soreness of the affected areas. Essential oils can soften the plugs inside the pores to ease their release—WITHOUT performing manual extractions. Check the formulas listed below for the ones for rosacea.

Aromatherapy Formulas for Cleansing Acne Skin

Formula #1: Use the baby bottle warmer. Place the sterile glass beaker inside and start by adding: 1 drop bergamot, 4 drops lavender, 2 drops juniper, and 1 drop rosemary. Stir until mixed. Then slowly add the 2 oz. of the base (which is the Aromatherapy Cleansing Formula #3 found in chapter 7, page 100.)

This is rather mild in comparison to other acne cleansers.

Formula #2: Follow steps for using baby bottle warmer. Start by adding: 8 drops palmarosa, 2 drops peppermint, and 4 drops sandalwood. Stir until mixed. Then slowly add the 2 oz. of the base—Cleansing Formula #3, page 100.

A unique blend of perky and woodsy. Popular with younger clientel.

Formula #3: Follow steps for using baby bottle warmer. Start by adding: 4 drops clary sage, 4 drops lemon oil and 4 drops violet leaf oil. Stir until mixed. Then slowly add the 2 oz. of the base—Cleansing Formula #3, page 100.

The refreshing nature of this cleanser makes it a hit with most everyone.

Formula #4: Follow steps for using baby bottle warmer. Start by adding: 8 drops eucalyptus, 2 drops juniper, and 2 drops patchouli. Stir until mixed. Then slowly add the 2 oz. of the base—Cleansing Formula #3, page 100.

This formula leaves the skin with a peppy feeling. **CAUTION:** Not designed for those clients with sensitive acne skin and/or pregnant.

A partial list of the essential oils known to be effective for **acne facial skin** includes: bergamot, carrot, chamomile, cypress, eucalyptus, geranium, hyssop, juniper, lavender, lemon oil, neroli, palmarosa, patchouli, peppermint, petitgrain, rosemary, sage, sandalwood, spearmint, tree tea, thyme, and violet leaf oil.

Aromatherapy Tonic Formulas for Acne Skin

> ### CAUTION
> When applying skin tonics, always shake the mixture thoroughly, and always cover the client's eyes before spraying.

Formula #1: Mix 3 oz. witch hazel with 1 oz. St. Johns Wort, and add: 8 drops patchouli, 4 drops clary sage, and 4 drops palmarosa. Put into a sprayer bottle.

This tonic is refreshing. It has a large, wide-ranging popularity.

Formula #2: Start with 4 oz. witch hazel and add: 2 drops bergamot and 5 drops thyme. Put into a sprayer bottle.

This tonic is not for the meek or timid. It packs a nice tingle.

> ### NOTE
> Refrigerate all tonic mixtures when not in use.

Rosacea Acne Skin Tonic: Formula #1: Mix 3 oz. witch hazel with 1 oz. cider vinegar and add: 2 drops bergamot and 8 drops clary sage. Put into a sprayer bottle.

This does the work without leaving a tremendous impact. Care must be taken with later exposure to the sun!

Moisturizing Acne Skin

The biggest mistake that clients and professionals make is to think that acne skin does not need moisture. It does not need any more oil, but for it to truly get under control, the water level must be put back on track. The following recipes will help solve this problem.

Aromatherapy Formulas for Moisturizing Acne Skin

Stage One

Acne Skin Formula #1: Start with 1 oz. lemon juice and add: 2 drops eucalyptus and 8 drops clary sage. Blend together and massage on clean skin for 5–8 minutes.

Mild but refreshing.

Formula #2: Start with 1 oz. almond oil and add: 1 drop bergamot, 4 drops calendula, and 4 drops lavender. Blend together and massage on clean skin for 5 minutes.

This has an unusual floral bouquet for an acne skin moisturizer. Female clients experiencing overly active skin in their late thirties and forties, love this one.

Formula #3: Start with 1 oz. evening primrose oil and add: 4 drops carrot, 4 drops palmarosa, and 4 drops yarrow. Blend together and massage on clean skin for 5 minutes.

This formula is especially appealing to men.

Formula #4: Start with 1 oz. borage seed oil and add: 8 drops myrrh, 4 drops rose and 4 drops chamomile. Blend together and massage on clean skin for 5 minutes.

First, check the client's reaction to myrrh. If positive, they will adore this mixture.

Stage Two

Acne Skin Formula #1: Start with 1 oz. almond oil and add: 5 drops chamomile, 20 drops carrot, and 3 drops calendula. Blend together and massage on clean skin for 5 minutes.

This formula fools the user. It is not as light-weight as others have been, but it really does work very well.

Formula #2: Start with 1 oz. evening primrose oil and add: 2 drops bergamot, 4 drops lavender, and 4 drops geranium. Blend together and massage on clean skin for 5 minutes.

The uniqueness of this blend creates an exotic aura. Many notice a calming effect very early in its usage.

Formula #3: Start with 1 oz. borage seed oil and add: 10 drops clary sage, 5 drops thyme, and 3 drops eucalyptus. Blend together and massage on clean skin for 5 minutes.

This has a punch to it that the hearty will enjoy and the timid will find harsh.

Stage Three

Acne Skin Formula #1: Start with 1 oz. almond oil and add: 4 drops neroli, 2 drops fennel and 4 drops parsley. Blend together and massage on clean skin for 5 minutes.

This is a real hit with anyone who loves to be outdoors. It's perfect for active clients.

Formula #2: Start with 1 oz. evening primrose oil and add: 10 drops juniper, 5 drops violet leaf, and 5 drops orange. Blend together and massage on clean skin for 5 minutes.

A mild formulation, it has an overall appeal due to its middle-of-the-road reaction to the nose.

Formula #3: Start with 1 oz. borage seed and add: 8 drops lavender, 8 drops geranium, and 8 drops rose. Blend together and massage on clean skin for 5 minutes.

This floral bouquet will appeal to the older clients who are still battling with their skin and the amount of water they are willing to drink.

Stage One

Rosacea Acne Skin Formula #1: Start with ½ oz. of chamomile and ½ oz. of almond oil and add: 6 drops parsley and 6 drops carrot. Blend together. Then use gentle, small, kneading massage movements over the affected areas.

The first impression about this formula may be that it seems too oily. However, like molecules bind and this formula will help lift the plugs out of the pores.

Formula #2: Start with 1 oz. chamomile and add 30 drops parsley. Blend together. Then use gentle, small, kneading massage movements over the affected areas.

This is a very mild formula that reduces redness. Clients love its action.

Stage Two

Rosacea Acne Skin Formula #1: Start with ½ oz. almond oil and ½ oz. aloe vera juice and add: 10 drops cypress and 10 drops geranium.

Blend together. Then use gentle, small, kneading massage movements over the affected areas.

The first impression about this formula may be that it seems to be too oily, it is not. Once the client gets use to the texture, they are impressed with its purging effect. Again the geranium makes it a huge hit.

Formula #2: Start with 1 oz. aloe vera juice and add: 5 drops cypress, 5 drops geranium, and 5 drops violet leaf. Blend together. Then use gentle, small, kneading massage movements over the affected areas.

This formula has similar reactions to those in Formula #1, above.

A partial list of the essential oils known to be effective for **rosacea facial skin** includes: bergamot, carrot, chamomile, cypress, geranium, hyssop, juniper, lavender, neroli, palmarosa, parsley, patchouli, rosewood, sage, spearmint, tree tea, thyme and violet leaf.

Aromatherapy Mask Formulas for Purging Acne/Oily Skin

Refer to the instructions for creating "Clay Mask Base Formula," page 117, to prepare the base for the following formulas.

Formula #1: Start with the base. Add: 3 drops eucalyptus, 1 drop peppermint, and 1 drop thyme. Blend well. Apply over the face with a fan brush. Leave on the skin for 5–7 minutes. Remove with a warm towel. (Preheat towels in a crockery cooking pot. Then they are ready anytime.) Spray the skin with an oily skin tonic.

This mask has a wonderful kick to it.

Formula #2: Start with the base. Add: 1 drop bergamot, 3 drops juniper, and 3 drops lemon oil. Follow the same application technique as mentioned above in Formula #1.

This mask is a lot milder than Formula #1, but still has a bit of a kick to it.

Formula #3: Start with the base. Add: 5 drops petitgrain, 5 drops sandalwood, and 5 drops patchouli. Follow the same application technique as mentioned in Formula #1.

The woodsy fragrance is appealing to men and outdoors-oriented women.

Formula #4: Start with the base. Add: 8 drops lavender, 8 drops juniper, and 6 drops thyme. Follow the same application technique as mentioned above in Formula #1.

This formula has a mild tingle due to the thyme. It has a wonderful unique blend that leaves the skin feeling alive.

A partial list of the essential oils known to be effective for **pulling masks for acne/oily facial skin** includes: bergamot, eucalyptus, juniper, lavender, lemon oil, palmarosa, patchouli, peppermint, petitgrain, rosemary, sandalwood, thyme, and violet leaf oil.

Chapter 9

Nail Care Formulas and Recipes

> *This section covers all aspects of manicuring services in the beauty industry. Details on basic hand and foot care are provided. Specific issues relating to nail care, as it pertains to currently followed procedures, are discussed. A detailed comparison between aromatherapy versus the conventional method of treatments used in the salon, is offered. Specific formulas are listed for both aromatherapy manicure and pedicure.*

Nail Condition and Appearance

Strong, healthy nails do not begin with the edge of the nails that get trimmed. You must begin with the area that is still continually alive. The nail bed and the cuticle are where you can make significant changes to improve the quality of the nails. Many physical conditions show up in the nails that are signals that medical attention is needed.

Arthritis and psoriasis are just two medical diseases that show up in the nails. Ridges and nail thickening are the two most often seen signals. A lifting of the nail bed is a sign of psoriasis. Only a medical doctor or trained practitioner can offer assistance. The manicurist can help the client to seek the proper attention, if they notice the condition when working on their client's nails.

It is the duty of every manicurist to thoroughly examine the nails of any customer, **before any service begins.** If a client is using artificial nails, the signals are more difficult to notice, so the manicurist should look at the nails before starting to do the full set. Obviously, it is very difficult to examine the nails of the client coming in with artificial nails already on, and requesting a fill. Even if the manicurist suggests that a new set be put on, the nails will be so very thin and fragile anyway. The manicurist should be on alert to see if the client's nails are experiencing a lot of lifting. A medical examination is definitely called for if there is lifting. You will gain the respect of the doctor and client alike, if you are the one to direct the client to seek the proper care.

Manicures

From the turn of the century, very wealthy men would get their nails "spit and polish" treatments at the town barber shop, along with a shave and a haircut. Starting in the seventies, it became acceptable for men to walk into full service salons and get their nails done while getting a haircut. Now in the nineties, manicures are not gender selective. With the increase of nail salons, male clients are just part of the clientele base.

A person's handshake says a lot about them in business. In fact so much so, that seminars dealing in personal development cover the topic. Therefore, manicurists are able to provide a valuable service to millions of professional business people. With the popularity of nail tips and acrylic nails, women are not getting manicures like they used to. Every two weeks they go to the nail salons for their fills. Aromatherapy can not really aid the manicurists with artificial nail services. It is incredibly useful in manicures, specifically with "hot oil manicures." The basis for aromatherapy treatments are the various essential oils. These oils have the power to penetrate deep into the skin. They have the ability to regenerate the skin tissue quicker than any standard hand cream, lotion, or oil. Using essential oils in the manicuring process will make an improvement in the client's hands on the very first treatment.

Just like any other part of the beauty industry, the need to stay competitive will be the driving force behind offering aromatherapy manicures. In California, it seems there are nail salons in every strip center, on every corner intersection. These nail salons are growing in number by the week. With so many to choose from, the need to offer more services is an obvious reality. Aromatherapy manicures will not take any more time than a standard manicure takes. It is the manicurist's decision how long they spend on each client. The area that makes the greatest impact is the massage time.

Standard Manicure

Supplies Needed

One manicure table	Cotton
One light/lamp source	Brand new orangewood sticks
One heater for oils or creams	Brand new nail file

Individual plastic liners for the heater

Rubbing alcohol (70% isopropyl alcohol)

Sterilized finger bath

Full selection of nail polishes

Sterilized nail clippers

Nail polish remover

Sterilized cuticle scissors

Cuticle remover lotion/cream

Sterilized nail brush

Hand cream

Roll of paper towels

Procedure

1. The manicurist or the client removes the nail polish with saturated cotton.
2. Rinse the nails to remove any remover residue.
3. One hand's nails are placed in warm water in the finger bath, while
4. On the other hand cuticle remover is applied to the nail beds to loosen dead skin off the nails. An orangewood stick is wrapped in cotton to clean under the nail beds, and then used to push off the cuticle skin that has been prepped by the cuticle remover.

   (Some manicurists will trim the cuticle tissue with clippers, however, the torn tissues called "hang nails" are easily created by this process. In many cases where the cuticles are clipped rather than worked with a cuticle pusher, "hang nails" show up the very next day. If you are a manicurist with the ability to work the cuticle clippers without this result, I take my hat off to you!)
5. The edges of the nails are then tapered with the file.
   The same series of processes are done on the other hand.
6. The hands and nails are placed in pre-warmed hand cream.
7. The manicurist massages the client's forearm, wrist and full hand.
8. Wipe away excess cream with alcohol.
9. Apply nail polish (base coat, color, and top coat), if desired.

Various massage movements can be utilized. Most often used is a version of **effleurage**, with a mild kneading action on the forearm. The wrist and digits are rotated and each gently tugged on. The palms are kneaded with the thumbs. The hand cream is used more for slippage during massage than chosen for its revitalizing capabilities. Often the excess is just wiped off. Although it does vary with each manicurist, the standard amount of time to massage BOTH arms, wrists, and hands averages under six minutes. Alcohol is used to remove the cream from the nails so the polish will be able to adhere properly. The nails are polished with base coat, color, and top coat. The standard manicure is completed.

Creating the Perfect Aromatherapy Manicure

The major differences between a standard manicure and an aromatherapy manicure are that in an aromatherapy manicure:

1. You can customize the oils used in the massage.
2. You are able to create a mixture that will bring about an immediate change in the appearance of the skin.
3. The attention to the client's skin is equal to the time spent on the nails.
4. A physical change in the client's hands are not just in the appearance of the polish on the nails.

Supplies Needed

One manicure table

One light/lamp source

One heater for oils or creams (A baby bottle warmer works great for aromatherapy formulations)

Individual plastic liners for the heater

Cotton

Brand new orangewood sticks

Brand new nail file

Sterilized finger bath

Sterilized nail clippers

Sterilized cuticle scissors

Sterilized nail brush

Roll of paper towels

Full selection of nail polishes

Rubbing alcohol (70% isopropyl alcohol)

Nail polish remover

Separate trolley (to hold all the essential oils, beakers, baby bottle warmer)

Essential oils

The process to take care of the edges of the nails will be the same as in the standard manicure. Although the manicurist will perform the cuticle removal technique, the solution for the cuticle removal is not a chemically prepared product. An aromatherapy formula works just as nicely.

If the client happens to have any fungus around the cuticle base, you can custom design the cuticle remover to adjust to the fungal infection. Clients whose hands are in frequent contact with water will most likely have a problem with fungus when wearing artificial nails. The long-term solution to the fungal infection problem is cosmetically the hardest one: remove the artificial nails and let the nail beds breathe. The client may cringe at having to deal with weak nails and not having the ten perfect looking nails. But if the fungus is not put under control and rid of totally, the end result will be NO NAILS at all. When this is put into the plainest of terms, the client will make the right choice.

With an aromatherapy manicure, the main difference falls in the conditioning of the skin and nail beds. The essential oils are used to create perfect formulations for each and every client. Small amounts of product is used, so there is virtually no waste. In addition, the fragrances that the essential oils emit into the air, aid in making the offensive smells of the acrylic powders less powerful.

In some formulations the natural fragrances can neutralize the offensive acrylic smells. Some nail salons use the natural fragrances of aromatherapy at the front door, so their clients have a positive experience walking in. The client's nose adjusts to the smell as they sit inside, though the first few seconds can be quite unpleasant. Smokers will be less sensitive to the natural aromas than nonsmokers.

Front-door fragrances can at the same time work against your treatment, if you are trying to use the essential oils to relax your customers. Experiment with the different blends of essential oils when you are using them in a small nail salon. You can create either a wonderful atmosphere, or one that causes the client to get agitated.

There are 17 vegetable bases (carrier oils), as listed on page 28, that can be mixed with the essential oils. Following is the list of the most commonly used essential oils in the nail industry. The successful manicurist will have all of these available for use in creating the perfect formula for each and every client.

1. Benzoin   4. Chamomile
2. Bois de rose   5. Clary sage
3. Carrot   6. Cypress

7. Fennel	17. Orange
8. Frankincense	18. Palmarosa
9. Geranium	19. Patchouli
10. Hyssop	20. Peppermint
11. Jasmine	21. Petitgrain
12. Juniper	22. Rose
13. Lavender	23. Rosemary
14. Lemon	24. Sandalwood
15. Marjoram	25. Ylang-Ylang
16. Neroli	

The manicurists must work together as a team, from one work station to another, to insure all of the clients sensitivities are taken into account. In most nail salons, since a close working relationship is developed amongst the staff and the regulars of the salon, learning the key allergic and/or sensitivities of each client will be quicker than in a full service style salon.

Begin all formulations with a base oil. Any one of the 17 previously mentioned will work. If you plan to massage both forearms and hands, a full two ounces are necessary. For only the hands and fingers, only one-half ounce will do just fine. It is better to need to mix more than waste the formula by having too much left over.

The following is an all-purpose formula that works well for any massage needs. Due to its versatility, the manicurist should make a full day's supply and keep it in a darkened glass bottle with a flip-top lid for easy access.

Aromatherapy All-Purpose Massage Oil

Single dosage

Formula #1: Using a baby bottle warmer, pre-heat 2 oz. of wheat-germ oil and add: 10 drops cypress, 10 drops neroli, and 10 drops orange. Stir well.

Pour only a portion of the solution into your palms and begin to massage the client's forearm, hand and fingers. Use standard **effleurage** manipulations. Work over the client's skin with your fingertips; NEVER use your nails. Depending on the client's health, the formula will either immediately melt into the skin, or it will take a few moments to penetrate. This formula offers wonderful viscosity, so your fingers should glide over the client's arms and hands very nicely.

Full day's supply

Formula #1: Use a sterile glass bottle with a flip-top lid for easy access. Start with 8 oz. of wheatgerm oil and add: 1 tbsp. cypress, 1 tbsp. neroli and 1 tbsp. orange. Stir briskly. Store away from direct light.

Use the same way as you would in individual Formula #1, above. This is just one very universal formula that any manicurist can create to use during the massage portion of the manicure service.

Although it makes sense to have a premade supply to accommodate hectic schedules, it is worth noting that part of the mystique and excitement from using aromatherapy in the salon is—for the client—the thrill of watching the formulations being created on-the-spot. This is why it is recommended that you have a special cart with wheels to hold all the bottles and materials to be blended. The cart can be wheeled up to each nail station, as needed, and all the other clients get to watch as the manicurist concocts the formula for the service. It is important for the manicurist to understand what can be offered to the client and what are just "happy but wishful-thinking ideas." An example of a first-time client manicure follows.

Sample Scenario: A First-Time Client's Aromatherapy Manicure

Mrs. Smith comes into a nail salon for the very first time. She made her appointment over the phone, and the receptionist asked her to come in for her first appointment without any nail polish on her nails. It is explained to her that the manicurist will review her nails before any chemicals are applied around her skin and nails. Before she is seated in the waiting area, a file card is provided for her to fill out her name, address, and home and work telephone numbers. She is asked to record the last time she had a nail appointment and what service was provided. She is asked to list ANY ALLERGIES she may have to anything at all, and to list any medications she is currently taking, or has taken in the last 30 days.

The manicurist reviews the card while looking over the client's hands, nails, and fingers. This information allows the manicurist to better service Mrs. Smith, by taking into account any current conditions that would have a direct impact on the formulas created for her manicure. Reviewing her hands and nails reveals:

Mrs. Smith has not had any artificial nails in the last year. The nail beds have good, pink color. The size of each nail varies in length, with the left hand's being slightly longer overall than the right hand's. The nail edges are smooth, except her left thumb-nail is badly bitten off. The cuticles are overgrown, and a little thick. There is a solid callus on her right index finger. All of the nail beds and edges appear thin. Mrs. Smith complains that her nails are easy to break.

The trained manicurist surmises that the client is right-handed, and apparently gnaws at her left thumbnail while under stress. She does not go in for professional manicures on a regular basis, nor does she know how to maintain her cuticles at home. With the nail beds being a healthy pink color, and having no visible indicators that she smokes, it is a good assumption that her thin nails are hereditary and not a lifestyle choice. The manicurist suggests that a series of four weekly appointments be set up to condition her cuticles and get her nail strength to improve.

An aromatherapy manicure would be an excellent choice for Mrs. Smith. She has a lot of cuticle to push back, but having her soak her fingers until the skin loosens will only make the nails appear more fragile. Using a cuticle softener formula to massage into the nail beds and cuticles after a "quick three-minute soak" will get great results. The manicurist massages the cuticles, works the tissue under with a cotton-padded orangewood stick.

The manicurist then proceeds to create a nail-strengthening solution to work into the client's nail beds to offer support to her nails. This is allowed to penetrate as Mrs. Smith's forearms are massaged with another skin smoothing formula. Since Mrs. Smith does not have a history of coming into a nail salon, she is enticed and fascinated by the mixing of solutions right in front of her. She marvels at the idea that this manicure was specifically created just for her and her special needs.

For the callus on her right index finger, the cuticle softener is applied over it. Then a piece of gauze saturated with the same solution is wrapped over the callus for the entire time of the service. It is only removed before Mrs. Smith leaves the salon. To file the callus down would only make the area predisposed to creating a larger one. The manicurist cannot expect her to change the way she holds her writing tool. Gently suggesting it may only make her more sensitive to the problem.

(On her next visit, the manicurist can present her with a rubberized sleeve for her pen or pencil. These are sold at any office supply store. They are inexpensive and this gesture will have a positive effect on Mrs. Smith's feeling that the manicurist cares about her as a person. Ask any beauty professional who has been in the business at least five years and they will tell you that you become an important part of your client's lives. They will tell you the most personal information about themselves and their families.)

Since Mrs. Smith's nails are of uneven lengths, all of her nails should be shortened for uniformity. The manicurist makes a strong suggestion to use a clear base and top coat painted over the nails, preferring to leave the choice of a colored polish to after several visits have improved her nails and they are longer. However, if Mrs. Smith has her heart set on wearing a colored polish, the manicurist guides her into selecting a light pastel color—not frosted or red—that would look appropriate on tiny nails.

Before the base and top coats are applied, the nails are wiped down with the small end of the orangewood stick, wrapped in cotton that has been saturated with a tiny amount of alcohol. This is CAREFULLY swiped over the nail bed, making sure not to touch the cuticles. The alcohol removes the oil and allows the base and top coats to stick properly. BEFORE Mrs. Smith's nails are painted, she is asked to pay for the service (most clients write a check and would not want to have wet nails as they do so) and asked what day the next week would best fit her schedule for her next appointment. She is reminded that, ideally, she should make four weekly appointments to condition her cuticles and strengthen her nails.

If you were the manicurist in the above scenario, DO NOT appear "pushy" at this time, this should be a smooth transaction. Let her have one of your cards to call in for her next appointment, suggesting two different days that have more flexibility for her ease in scheduling. If there is any hesitation, try the following dialogue: "Here is my card, Mrs. Smith. Right now it appears that Wednesday afternoon and Friday morning are particularly flexible; please check your date planner and don't hesitate to give us a call to let us know what works best for you."

Should you be able to keep to a tight schedule without making your customers wait, you can add: "I even specialize in getting you in and out within a lunch-hour break, if that will work in your schedule too." This lets her know that she can depend on you to not keep her waiting. With all the hectic time restraints of career-minded people, this flexibility is a service that is particularly beneficial.

Suggesting four weekly appointments will appear less constricting than saying a full month's schedule. It gives the client the illusion of more control over the idea, and room to change the schedule to biweekly sessions, if four appointments are not acceptable.

It is important to remember the best laid plans will not work if not followed. New customers may seem to agree to anything presented at the time they are in the salon. Then, after they get home, they may change their minds entirely to the point of never returning. The professional manicurist must learn how to offer suggestions that appear to be what the customer wants right from the beginning. This is not easily accomplished but should be worked on over and over again, until it becomes a natural way of speaking. It would be a valuable investment in the beginning of your career, if you were to find a successful manicurist and offer to work for them for one month as their "nail polisher." In those 20 working days (or whatever time you could afford), you will get to see and hear how it is done, and get to pick up "tips-of-the-trade" that only comes from years of experience.

Aromatherapy Cuticle Softener Formulas

Formula #1: Lightly warm ½ oz. jojoba oil and mix into it: 2 drops eucalyptus and 5 drops carrot. Stir and begin to gently massage it into the cuticles. Using circular motions of your fingertips over each cuticle bed, spend up to one minute massaging each finger. Have ready at least two orangewood sticks pre-wrapped with cotton. You will use these sticks to lift the cuticle off the nail bed and to GENTLY ROLL the cuticle skin under. **CAUTION:** Do not cut the skin.

Formula #2: Preheat ½ oz. grapeseed oil and add: 5 drops lemon, and 2 drops peppermint. Stir and follow the same massage and instructions as in Formula #1, above.

Aromatherapy Hand Cream Formulas

Creating a base will make customizing the hand cream easier and less time-consuming than making all of it on an "as needed" basis. The base can be stored in the refrigerator in a sealed container.

This formula requires one full stick of all-natural cocoa butter. (You can find cocoa butter in sticks at any health food store or naturalist store.) You need to melt the cocoa butter down into a soft, pliable blob. A baby bottle warmer works well, as will a carefully monitored microwave oven. You can even use a double boiler, if you want to make it at home and then bring it in to work. The cocoa butter needs to be squishy like very soft butter, BUT NOT LIQUIFIED. After melting 1 stick cocoa butter, add: 4 tsp. almond oil. Stir until blended. This is the base.

Place the mixture in a sterile glass jar. Keep the lid tight when not using it. Storing it in the refrigerator will require you to reheat small amounts of the base as needed. If you are working in a large nail salon, this base can be used up every day. In place of the almond oil, you can use any of the 17 base/carrier oils for this base, and the selection can be based on the client's fragrance preferences. Of course, any client allergies should be the main criteria for this decisions making.

Using the base, you can add up to any 10 drops of the essential oil(s) of your liking. You can split the ten drops into two 5-drop concentrations or any other combination of ten to your suiting. The solutions are endless. You can be adventurous with the essential oils and try all of them.

Here are just some examples of possible hand creams:

Formula #1: Preheat 1 heaping tbsp. of the base to soften, and add: 2 drops carrot, 2 drops geranium, 2 drops patchouli, and 2 drops sandalwood. Stir until completely mixed. Use deep tissue massage movements to penetrate the solution into both hands and wrists.

Formula #2: Start with 1 heaping tbsp. preheated and softened base and add: 5 drops neroli and 5 drops lemon. Stir and perform the same massage movements as in Formula #1, above.

Formula #3: Start with the same base and add: 3 drops lavender, 2 drops rosemary, and 4 drops carrot. Follow instructions found in Formula #1, above.

Formula #4: Again use the warmed base and add: 8 drops evening primrose and 2 drops peppermint. Follow the same instructions as in Formula #1.

Aromatherapy Formulas for Oil-Based Massage Solutions

Some clients will come in for a manicure, and in an instant you will see that their skin has really been challenged. For these manicures, use an oil solution for massaging.

Formula #1: Using a heater, pour 1 oz. avocado oil and add: 2 capsules vitamin E (puncture each gel cap and squeeze the fluid into the mixture), 6 drops carrot, and 5 drops geranium. Stir well and use deep tissue massage movements to penetrate the solution into the client's hands and wrists.

Formula #2: Use the same heater, pour ½ oz. of almond oil and ½ oz. of jojoba oil and add: 20 drops evening primrose and 10 drops sandalwood. Stir well. Massage deeply into the client's hands and wrists.

Formula #3: Preheat 1 oz. grapeseed oil and add: 1 capsule vitamin E (puncture and empty into the mixture), 5 drops rose, and 5 drops lavender. Stir and use as described in Formula #1 above.

When mixing the essential oils into the selected base oil, start with 10 as the total number of drops to add. Gently warm all of the oils. They'll blend better and massage more easily into the skin and nails. The more advanced manicurist can create endless combinations of manicuring oils.

Aromatherapy is not just for customizing the massage vehicle or making the potion for the cuticles during the manicure. It can help improve the health of the client's nails, arms, and hands. The average clients subject their hands to rough work, strong chemicals, and frequent washings every day. This abuse is a necessary part of living, and few people can find ways to change their daily lifestyle to help reduce their hands taking such rough treatment. Therefore, the manicurist that can offer solutions to these harsh realities of life, will have clients coming back for as long as they stay in business. Aromatherapy is the key to success.

Chapter 10

Specific Nail Conditions and Formulas

> *This section explores some of the most popular problems facing the average client. Holistic explanations are provided on the reasons for the conditions and what can be done to improve them.*

Brittle Nails and Cuticles

Brittle cuticles tear easily and the clients with these usually complain of constant "hangnails." Hangnails (agnails) are thin slivers of skin hanging around the nails. Many people can't resist the temptation to pull, or even bite, these pieces of skin off. The areas around the back of the nail beds usually look raw and unsightly. Minor infections are also more likely to occur if the client tears these skin tags off themselves.

The manicurist should ask the client if they have received manicures in the recent past during which the cuticles were clipped off. This clipping technique for cuticle removal promotes hangnails, too. Read the information in the standard manicuring section (page 136), for the proper method to care for cuticles. After cuticle remover is used, aromatherapy oil can be massaged into the area.

If the client complains that they have always had problems with cracking and tearing of the cuticle area, ask questions to determine if any of the following are factors: diet, level of water intake, heredity and/or life-style choices such as exposing their hands to harsh chemicals.

If their diet is the main reason, the aromatherapy formulas will offer nutrients to the skin for balance. You can create a special aromatherapy solution, that the client can purchase for homecare use at night.

Brittle nails can be caused by internal, systemic conditions. Most often it stems from part of the client's family genetic coding. Although drinking sufficient amounts of water would be helpful, it is not the only solution. Brittle nails are usually thin and fragile. Brittle nails are usually accompanied by brittle cuticles, but not necessarily vice versa. They will split, crack, and break without too much force being put upon the nails. Aromatherapy can have a positive impact on these nails.

There are several factors to consider when determining if a positive change in the condition is realistic:

- The severity of the condition.
- How long the condition has gone on untreated.
- How dedicated the client is to protecting the nails from outside conditions, i.e. harsh chemicals, long hours at a keyboard or typewriter, heavy manual labor.

This condition often results in the manicurist offering to put arcylic nails or silk wraps over the brittle nails. The idea is by covering it over you will not have to deal with the condition. However, brittle nails are not truly strong enough to be good candidates for artificial nails or the strong adhesive used in silk wraps. The decision to put acrylic nails or silk wraps over these nails should be put off until after 90 days of dedicated effort working on improving them is completed. If, at the end of the 90 days, a significant improvement is not offered, then applying the acrylic nails or silk wraps seems an appropriate choice.

Brittle nails sometimes have ridges over the nail bed. If so, ask if the client has recently had artificial nails removed. The ridges may be a sign of uneven drill work. If they have, in fact, had that done within the last six months, recommend that they make weekly appointments with you to treat the nails and cuticles to return the nails to a smooth texture. This will take at least three months of continual care to reduce the damage the drilling created. It may be very difficult to have the client understand and appreciate all the time and effort it will take to undo the damage. So often clients want a "quick fix" and the truth is, none exists.

Part of the solution to aiding a client with a hereditary disposition to brittle nails, is to suggest they eat a well-balanced diet, with plenty of vitamins. Calcium is a mineral that is a very important factor in growing strong nails. Some believe eating gelatin for its keratin will help. It will not hurt anything, but the increase in keratin is so very minor, that it's help to brittle nails is not noticeable.

Another part of the treatment of brittle nails is the increase in oxygen to the base of the nail bed. The edge of the nail is the only part that is completely dead. The nail directly under the cuticle area is where most of the improvement will take place, since this is the area that is still very much alive and thriving. The lunula, commonly referred to as the "half-moon" is also very much alive. The keratin fibers of the nail are nourished in these two areas. Any signs of damage will first be seen in and around the lunula.

The keratin fibers of the nail are 50 times more tightly woven than those found in the skin. As in all hereditary factors, we get what we have been born with in the thickness of the keratin weave. No one can change the biological thickness of the skin to be more than when we were born. The same is not true with the keratin fibers of the nails.

Following certain lifestyle choices, including the diet we keep, a change in the thickness of the nails can be brought about, but only within a set range. The nails can only change by a percentage of the basics given at birth. Ask the client if their parents both had brittle nails. This will give you an idea of the gene-pool from which the client's nails are based.

NOTE

Pre-natal vitamins were not used as extensively as they are now. If your client is over 40, they may not have had the added nutrients that pregnant mothers get today. Should your client be one of a multiple birth, such as twins, their nails may be calcium deficient from birth, too. Client's history does have an impact on their future nails.

Lifestyle choices, like not eating vegetables other than potatoes, will have a negative effect on brittle nails. The amount of caffeine ingested will also impede the improvement of brittle nails. This includes coffee, tea, and sodas. Cigarette smoking also makes nails more brittle, since tar and nicotine end up in the keratin fibers of our hair, skin, and nails. No amount of aromatherapy can undo the damage of a smoker. Realize what you are up against, before making any claims for improvement!

Whether the condition is serious or mild, aromatherapy formulas provide at least temporary assistance to the appearance of frail, brittle nails. After treatment, they will look smooth and shiny, with a marked increase in natural coloring under the nails. The aromatherapy formulas offer an increase in blood flow to the fingertips and under the nails. In some formulas there will be a warming sensation deeper than that coming from the heated oil. Vasodilation causes an inner heat the client will sense very quickly. This is normal. For sensitive clients, it is best to let them know in advance that the "inner warming" is ok.

CAUTION

Special care must be practiced when using specific oils.

Remember: Rosemary, sage, eucalyptus, hyssop, fennel, and tagetes (among others) are **very dangerous** to pregnant women.

Eucalyptus and lemongrass **cannot** be used on young children.

Bergamot is **very dangerous** to any client with photo-sensitivity.

Aromatherapy Formulas for Brittle Nails and Cuticles

Formula #1: Warm 3 tbsp. of evening primrose oil and add: 3 drops eucalyptus. Stir, and gently dip a cotton swab into the oil. Distribute the oil around the cuticle beds on each finger. Then using circular motions, massage each cuticle bed with your thumb pad. Spend around one minute massaging each finger (allow approximately 10 minutes for this step). After working on both hands, go back to the first finger and GENTLY PUSH the cuticle skin under the bed, using a cotton-covered orangewood stick. After working all cuticle beds, massage the remaining oil into the entire nail beds of each finger. Re-dip the cotton swab, and coat UNDER each nail's free edge.

This formula will produce a very slight warming sensation as you work it into the cuticle skin and over the brittle nail beds. The increased circulation offers an improvement to the natural coloring of the nail bed. **CAUTION:** Not for pregnant women.

Formula #2: Warm 3 tbsp.avocado oil and add: 2 drops carrot, 6 drops peppermint, and 8 drops lemon oil. Stir. Follow the same application instructions as in Formula #1, above.

This formula will also produce a warming sensation. The lemon makes the coloring of the nail bed even clearer. This formula will be wonderful for a smoker with yellowy nail beds.

Formula #3: Warm 3 tbsp. grapeseed oil and add: 4 drops eucalyptus and 4 drops peppermint. Follow the application instructions found in Formula #1.

Since two vasodilaters are being introduced to the cuticles and nail beds, every strong inner heat sensation will be noticeable.

Formula #4: Warm 3 tbsp. jojoba oil and add: 10 drops lemon, 6 drops carrot, and 6 drops cypress. Stir. Follow the application instructions found in Formula #1.

This formula is mild in comparison to the others. There should not be any sensation from the application. For nails that are really thin and fragile, as well as brittle, this formulation will be easier to handle.

Rough, Coarse, Skin-damaged Hands

Although severely conditioned hands are the biggest challenge, the clients with these hands are also likely to become the most loyal customers, if you can turn their hands back to normal condition. You must get them to realize that lifestyle changes are probably needed. They have to change the way they wash their hands, the way they expose their hands to harsh chemicals. Also, the water temperature they use to shower or bathe in has to be reduced.

You can create a special formula that can be massaged into the hands to protect them from outside influences. These formulas will feel slippery and the clients will have to adjust their grips. One possible solution is to have clients wear gloves over their hands to protect the formula and provide better grip.

Intensive Aromatherapy Skin Protector Formulas

Formula #1: Use a double boiler or baby bottle warmer. Melt ½ stick cocoa butter, 4 tbsps. of beeswax (found in health food stores), and 1 oz. of apricot kernel. Slowly add: ½ tsp. borax, ½ cup distilled water, 8 drops lavender, 3 drops rosemary, and 2 drops thyme. Stir continuously. This solution will penetrate the skin on the hands if deeply massaged, but will also leave a film on the surface. Slow effleurage movements will work well. Remove the formula from the nails if intending to polish nails during service, as the formula will make polishing the nails impossible. To remove formula from nails, put alcohol on a cotton swab and work it over the nails. Put any leftover mixture in a sterile glass container with a tight lid, to store for future use.

This will be a favorite for many clients with hands that look as painful as they feel. The thyme will tingle but not very much.

Formula #2: Use a double boiler or baby bottle warmer. Melt 1 stick of cocoa butter, 1 heaping tablespoon of glycerine and 1 oz. of almond oil. Stir while you add: 10 drops patchouli. The mixture will leave a film on the skin's surface. Use the same application instructions as mentioned in Formula #1 above.

This formulation will be effective and mild to the skin. For any sensitive clients, choose this one.

Essential Oils Specific to Treatment of Hands, Nails, and Feet

For the professional manicurist with more advanced training in aromatherapy, following are partial lists of the essential oils that have healing properties for the hands, nails and feet. As always, CHECK FOR ALLERGIES BEFORE CREATING ANY FORMULATIONS. For a single application, begin with one teaspoon of a base/carrier oil (the 17 base/carrier oils are listed on page 28) and add any one of the essential oils to it. The total number of drops should fall into the 6–10 drop range, except when fighting fungi; judge those differently. Fungi-fighting formulas are listed later in this chapter.

Essential oils with healing properties for the hands include: Carrot, eucalyptus lemon, geranium, lavender, lemon, lime, neroli, palmarosa, rose, rosemary, and sandalwood.

Essential oils with healing properties for the nails include: Carrot, eucalyptus peppermint, eucalyptus radiata, grapefruit, lavender, lemon, myrrh, patchouli, oregano, rosemary, sandalwood, tea tree, tagetes, and thyme.

Essential oils with healing properties for the feet include: Calendula, carrot, chamomile, fennel, lavender, lemon, palmarosa, tagetes and thyme.

Damaged Nail Beds

Unlike in the condition of brittle nails, for which there can be genetic reasons and/or lifestyle causes, damaged nails are caused by definite human error. As of late, the most common cause is the drilling for acrylic nail fillings during nail appointments. Other causes are doing housework, home repairs, or working on cars, where tools like hammers, screwdrivers, or staple guns are used. It is common for people to take their hands and nails for granted, and so damage occurs. The good news is that the body is reasonably forgiving, and has the ability to repair itself. There are, however, some repairs that are not so easily corrected.

The Black Nail

Black nail is caused by direct force to the nail. The nail bed gets bruised so badly that it dies and turns black. Most often the capillaries in the soft tissue under the traumatized nail break, then clot, and the clot turns to a black color. With time, the clot will be re-absorbed and disappear. Time is needed to regrow another nail. Instead of weeks, it will take several months for the nail to grow out. The new nail will replace the dead one. Sometimes the nail bed will disattach itself from the skin underneath. The person must tend to and "baby" the nail so that it does not fall off prematurely (before the new nail has grown out). There can be conditions that will make the nail fall off too early. If the soft tissue under the nail bed swells too much with a large blood clot, it will lift the nail bed. Then when the clot gets reabsorbed , it leaves a significant gap where the nail bed cannot reattach itself and subsequently falls off.

Once the nail is dead and the blood clot is gone, the person should get to a professional manicurist for help. The manicurist can show them how to gently and very carefully massage the cuticle tissue of the nail. The cuticle area is where the new, fresh nail will come. The massage improves the area's oxygen transfer. The better the oxygen transfer, the healthier the cuticles and thus the greater the chance the nail has to come out in perfect condition. Refer to the aromatherapy formulas for improvement of cuticles earlier in this chapter. These formulas will aid these damaged cuticles too.

Drill Bit Grooves

A client's nails may show ridges that are caused from the nail drill bit used to remove acrylic nails. Sometimes the natural nail is grazed by the nail drill used to remove the acrylic nails. It is very difficult for a manicurist to hold a drill so carefully that it only touches the acrylic nails and NOT the natural nail. Since the nails are being covered by the acrylic coating, there is a false sense of security that it does not make any difference what the natural nail look like. However, these ridges can make permanent scars that will remain over the nails, if repeated grazing is endured over time. The acrylic coatings can be soaked off and removed, the scars cannot. Sadly, aromatherapy cannot help the problem.

This text makes note of this condition because the professional manicurist has the option to use other methods to work the acrylic off of the nail bed, other than the drill, and it might be worth taking another look at these options. They include using a manual file or rough-grained buffing block, or using nippers to pick off the lifting parts of the acrylic nail.

Split/Cracked Nails

If the free edge of the nail gets a crack, a nail file or emery board can quickly remedy the problem. However, if the crack works itself down to the attached portion of the nail, a more serious problem develops. The crack or separation creates a pattern for the nail to continue as it moves forward.

The free edge portion of the nail is the only part of the nail that is truly dead. As the nail grows under the cuticles, the free edge is pushed forward. Left alone, the nail grows quite lengthy. It is dead tissue with no connection to the healthy nail. If the crack is part of the new nail growth, than the dead portion will have a continuous crack in it. No amount of filing the free edge will help. If the client seeks professional help from a manicurist in time, the course of the damage can be changed.

Treatment

First, the manicurist files the free edge down close to the top of the connected nail. Second, the the crack is gently buffed down to become smooth and even. Next, a series of massage manipulations are performed to increase the blood flow to the area. The natural process of nutrients getting to the weakened area through the blood flow will give the nail a fighting chance to repair itself.

Aromatherapy is an effective tool in getting nutrients to the spot through vasodilation. Applying the oils and massaging the nail will take just a few moments. This treatment **must** be repeated several times a day for at least one week. Therefore, the manicurist should teach the client how to use the formula at home before retiring at night, and again in the morning. Although probably not practical, it would be even more beneficial to repeat the treatment at least once during the day. Perhaps suggest to the client to do it over a lunch break, since it will take less than one minute to complete.

Aromatherapy Vasodilation Formulas

Formula #1: Using a heater pot or baby bottle warmer, LIGHTLY warm 1 teaspoon sesame oil and add: 2 drops eucalyptus and 1 drop thyme. Stir. Dip a cotton swab into the oil and apply it directly on the nail where the crack had been. Next roll the slightly dampened cotton swab underneath the free edge, concentrating near the connecting area. Then in circular movements, manipulate your thumb over the entire nail bed to increase the blood flow.

The sesame oil is rich in Vitamin E, and the thyme and eucalyptus will cause a cool heat sensation. The coloring under the nail will flush.

Other variations will provide the same vasodilation. If the client finds the smell of eucalyptus is too medicinal, substitute peppermint for the eucalyptus. Also, you can split the two drops to 1 peppermint and 1 eucalyptus. Always include the thyme. The one teaspoon will last for several applications.(5–7 treatments).

For one week usage, increase the mixture to the following: Start with 1 tablespoon of sesame oil and add: 8 drops eucalyptus (or split it 4 peppermint and 4 eucalyptus) and 4 drops thyme.

Ingrown Nails

Sometimes clients mention that their mom or grandmother had ingrown nails. This condition could possibly have hereditary patterns to it. What is more likely to have been passed down through the generations is the way clients are taught to cut their nails. Ingrown nails are most often created by improper nail trimming. The large toe nails are the most common nails to become ingrown. Poorly fit, or too tight, shoes can cause the condition, too.

Nail trimming should be left to the professional. Clients seldom attempt to cut their own hair, they leave that job for their hairdresser or barber. They should leave the job of trimming their nails to the manicurist. If they cannot or will not, there are some guidelines the professional can offer.

The nails should be clean and softened. At-home nail trimming should be done immediately after a bath or shower. Leaving at least ¼ inch of free edge from the connecting nail tissue is recommended. Cut straight across, and then use a nail file or emery board to finish the process. This eliminates creating the situation that promotes the ingrown nail.

If the nail is cut too close to the connecting tissue, pressure is created that forces the soft tissue to expand forward, thus forcing the nail to fold under the skin. As the nail attempts to grow forward, it is pushed into the soft tissue and is very painful.

To treat an ingrown nail, the manicurist has to perform the delicate task of lifting the nail up and over the skin. If the condition is too severe, the client must seek the help of a podiatrist. (Remember: When in doubt, send the client to a doctor!)

A small piece of cotton placed under the curved, ingrown nail will lift the nail and elevate the pressure. The skin will be very tender, red, and sore. Aromatherapy offers assistance in reducing the soreness.

Aromatherapy Calming Formulas for Tender, Red, and Sore Nail Areas

Formula #1: Begin by chilling one ounce Chinese tea and add: 10 drops chamomile and 10 drops patchouli. Blend. Saturate a cotton pad with the solution. Wrap around the sore nail for 15 minutes.

This solution will look almost good enough to drink. The nail will feel better and the redness is dramatically reduced.

Formula #2: Chill one ounce witch hazel and add: 10 drops yarrow and 10 drops violet leaf oil. Blend and follow the same application instructions as in Formula #1.

This mixture will appeal to men, too. The reactions will be similar to Formula #1.

Formula #3: Chill one ounce ginger root tea and add: 10 drops lavender and 10 drops tea tree. Blend and follow application instructions found in Formula #1.

This tea has a very oriental fragrance and is very popular amongst both men and women.

Fungus Growth

The most common of all fungus growth is ringworm, commonly called "athlete's foot." No matter what age group, gender, or activity, anyone can get it. It turns any area between the toes or fingers into swollen, itchy, flaky irritations. The skin often turns white and spongy, like being waterlogged. All it takes to get it is walking barefoot over the exact area that an infected person has just walked barefoot. One time that's all. Swimming pools, Jacuzzis (whirlpool baths), gyms, locker rooms, showers, and public bathrooms are classic areas for the fungus to breed.

If the fungus is left to grow, and it does so *very* quickly, all of your toes can become infected in a matter of days. Then, if toes are scratched to alleviate the itch, the fungus can get trapped under the fingernail(s) and spread to all of the fingers. Fungi are hearty and indiscriminate for hosts.

There are other kinds of fungi that are similar to the athlete's foot type. They grow due to trapped moisture under acrylic nail coatings or silk wraps. A slight lifting of the acrylic will allow a water or moisture droplet to seep underneath. This fungus grows quickly, too. Women who frequently have their hands in water are most susceptible to fungal growths. Removing the coating is an appropriate first step, but many do not. You can dip the nails in tincture of zinc and/ or white vinegar. Dry them thoroughly, afterward.

The good news is that the aromatherapy treatments are just as quick, and effective, as the over-the-counter medicines. Being freshly prepared, they can be whipped together in a minute's notice. The client won't have to keep old cans of medicine around. The aromas from these formulas are strong, although nicer than those of the typical over-the-counter antifungal sprays.

Aromatherapy Formulations for Attacking Fungus Growth

Foot Soak

Formula #1: To eliminate the itch and burning sensations. Pour very warm water (everyone has their own heat comfort level) into a large bowl or bucket, and add: one cup of salt (rock salt [kosher] works well, as does epsom salt.) Stir to dissolve. Then add: 8 drops tea tree, and 4 drops lavender. Stir by swishing the feet around in the water. Soak the feet for 10–15 minutes. Dry the feet very thoroughly.

Antifungal Formulations

Formula #1: Only a very small amount is needed. Mix 1 tsp. wheatgerm oil with 10 drops tea tree and 5 drops patchouli. Saturate a cotton swab and cover the infected areas. Put on latex gloves and massage the oil mixture deep into the skin. Apply this mixture to the infected areas daily, until the fungi are all gone. Instruct client to wear only very clean, white, 100% cotton socks.

Tea tree is very pungent, and most people will not find the aroma terribly appealing. Getting rid of the fungi condition, is worth it.

Formula #2: Mix 1 tsp. jojoba oil with 10 drops lemon oil and 15 drops tagetes. Wear latex gloves. Use a saturated cotton swab and cover the infected areas. Massage ointment into the skin. Apply daily until it is no longer needed. Instruct client to wear only clean, white, 100% cotton socks.

Tagetes is also unpleasant smelling. The lemon will cut some of the smell, as well as work off the dead, spongy skin cells.

Formula #3: Mix 1 tsp. sesame oil with 20 drops cypress, 4 drops thyme, and 10 drops tea tree. Use the cotton swab and gloves to apply and massage. Apply daily until the fungi are gone. Instruct client to wear only clean, white, 100% cotton socks.

The thyme and tea tree will make the skin tingle. It will be a refreshing change from the itchy, burning sensation caused by the fungus.

A partial list of the essential oils known to have **antifungal properties includes:** balsam de Peru, eucalyptus lemon, hyssop, juniper, lavender, lemon, melissa, myrrh, patchouli, pimiento, sage, sandalwood, sarriette, tagetes, tea tree, and thyme. When making the solution, consider how severe the fungus infection is, and how long it has been present. The formulation will go from very mild to strong. The number of drops to use with a teaspoon of base oil will range from 15–60 drops. There is no ironclad formula measure, you will have to judge each case separately. A very rough guide for measurement is as follows:

MILD: 15–25 drops   MODERATE: 25–40 drops
SEVERE: 40–60 drops

CAUTION

Always instruct the client to wear clean, white, 100% cotton socks. It may sound like simple common sense, but make sure the client knows not to wear the same socks more than once, after workouts, or any other reason. Nylon, acrylic blends, and polyester materials will not let the skin breathe like cotton does. Wool is the only other fiber to select for socks. Colored socks are forbidden, because the dye may enter the pores or open wounds, causing further discomfort or damage.

Chapter 11

Aromatherapy Pedicures

One of the most pampering services to be provided by a manicurist is the pedicure. Reputations are built faster from this service than any other one. It is, however, the one service that requires the most physical exertion. Many manicurists have negative feelings about doing them, although if done well, the clients adore them. The following sections detail the differences between standard and aromatherapy pedicures. Specific formulations are also provided.

Feet and Physical Condition

The feet are parts of the body that can carry many germs, fungus, and strong negative odors. Many women wear fashion shoes that ruin their feet. They come to the professional with hopes that a pedicure will undo the damage. In reality, an excellent pedicure can temporarily reduce and remove signs of shoe abuse. If the client is set on continuing to wear the shoes, the conditions return shortly.

Some calluses are caused by spinal problems. Bunions and bone spurs are definitely caused by improper balance of the spine, hips, and/or legs. Clients with these conditions MUST be referred to a doctor. A pedicure will not and cannot eliminate these conditions, although a release of pressure during the pedicure will lessen the discomfort or pain. (It is acceptable to have business cards for referrals to competent orthopedics, podiatrists, and chiropractors. Allowing clients to choose their own specialists will avoid any liability and/or perceived conflicts of interest.)

The professional pedicurist/manicurist must ask each new client some health questions BEFORE beginning the service. Depending on the answers, it may be necessary to forego any appointment. Some salons have the receptionist try to ask the questions over the phone, this is a poor choice. The relationship established for the future should be started with a face-to-face inquiry. If done over the phone, the potential client is left with the sense that they are not wanted.

Some general guidelines to follow to keep you from getting into trouble, as well as potentially saving the client from having a bad experience, are listed below.

Clients with High Blood Pressure

Strong caution should be taken with any client suffering from high blood pressure. Water temperatures have to be moderate. Special care must be taken not to cut their skin during the pedicure.

Clients with Diabetes

Diabetes is a disease that makes a pedicure a restricted treatment. Diabetes can cause the patient to lose their feet, therefore no service should be done without their physician's prior approval. The client can bleed very easily and the calluses can be extremely thick. Diabetics have a difficult time determining if hot water is too hot for their comfort. Always test the water before they place their feet into the tub or foot bath.

Clients with Cancer

Any form of skin cancer should be a signal not to do a pedicure. If the client is undergoing chemotherapy, no service should be completed without their physician's permission.

Clients Taking Medication

NO sharp instruments are to be used on the calluses of clients taking medication, such as a blood thinner, or aspirin. All efforts should be made to make sure that no bleeding occurs.

Pedicure Chair/Bath Types

The professional manicurist has the opportunity to offer several different kinds of pedicures to their clients. Some salons use simple, separate buckets or the plastic bucket-style foot baths with heaters and vibrating motors; while others use a sophisticated spa chair with whirlpool jets and full vibrating massage motors inside the chair.

The real quality in a pedicure should come from the techniques used, not from the bucket or chair. Much fuss and bother has been made over their differences. The spa chairs are very, very nice, but they can never replace the results obtained from the hands of a competent pedicurist/manicurist.

Check with your individual state boards of cosmetology for the restrictions and limitations regarding the supplies and equipment allowed. Many states prohibit razor-style instruments to be used to remove calluses.

Sterilization

With current medical conditions like AIDS, HIV, hepatitis (A, B, and C), and others; it is imperative that STRICT STERILIZATION be followed. As previously mentioned, it is important to get a medical history on every new client. Due to the rules protecting clients' privacy, some important information will not be easy to obtain. As precautions, disposable items should be selected, when possible, over other tools.

The salon should have several different kinds of sterilization tools available:

A wet sterilizer, using quats and other antiviral, antibacterial solutions.

Ultraviolet light cabinet to use overnight to sterilize instruments.

An autoclave is the best form of sterilization. This equipment is expensive, and special care is needed when operating it.

Standard Pedicure Equipment and Supplies

Supplies needed for the standard pedicure are about the same as the manicure:

One pedicure table/tray to hold supplies

One light/lamp source

One heater for oils or creams

Individual plastic liners for the heater

Cotton

Brand new orangewood sticks

Brand new nail file

Two sterilized foot baths (one for cleaning, one for rinsing), OR standard plastic foot bath with electric heater and vibrating motor; OR spa chair (with whirlpool jets and vibrating massage motors)

Sterilized nail clippers

Sterilized cuticle scissors

Sterilized nail brush

Roll of paper towels

Full selection of nail polishes

Alcohol (rubbing or 70% isopropyl alcohol)

Nail polish remover

Cuticle remover lotion/cream

Hand cream

Additional Equipment: Electric booties and a crockery cooking pot for dry, warmed towels (the pot would only require 3 oz. of water on the bottom.) In addition, the manicurist needs graters and sanders for the calluses and rough spots on the feet, especially around the heels.

NOTE

Remember, many states prohibit the use of razor devices like the Credo Knife. Check with your local authorities. Regardless, any razor blade tool, requires hands-on training, and a lot of it, before using on a client. A new blade must be used for every client, no exceptions.

Standard Pedicure Process

If possible, have the client come to the salon with open-toed shoes and pants that can roll up to the kneecaps. Once they arrive, have them pick out the polish color and get their feet ready to soak in the foot bath.

The manicurist has prepared a tray with all of the tools, towels, files, polish, etc., that will be needed during the pedicure. Setting up the tray ahead of time saves time, and allows the manicurist to have continuous contact with the client. For added convenience, some manicurists set the tub up right next to their manicuring table. However, unless a supportive, backed chair is also brought next to the manicuring table, the client is inconvenienced by having to sit in a small chair or stool. Avoid compromising the client's comfort for your convenience. Also, NEVER have the client lean up against the wall for support during a pedicure. It simply is not an option.

The bath is half-filled with warm water and 1 ounce of quaternary ammonium compounds (quats) disinfectant solution. (Again, check with your local state board of cosmetology regarding the regulations on sterilization.) The heat and vibration buttons are turned on, if using a whirlpool spa, and/or the client places their feet inside the bath.

Pre-Massage Procedure

1. Remove any toenail polish with a piece of cotton saturated with polish remover.
2. Rinse the toes to remove any residue, by re-dipping them into the foot bath.
3. With one foot still soaking in the bath, apply cuticle remover to the other toenails to loosen the dead skin off of the nails.
4. Wrap an orangewood stick in cotton to clean under the nail beds.
5. Work off the cuticle skin that has been prepped by the cuticle remover. (Some manicurists will trim the cuticle tissue with clippers, however, the torn tissue called hangnails are easily created by this process. If you have the ability to work the cuticle clippers without this result, my hat is off to you!
6. File the edges of the toe nails straight across with a file.

Pedicure Massage

Now the massage begins. The massage can be a real delight to perform and to receive. This is the real part of the pedicure that makes or breaks the service. Many manicurists rush through this part for various reasons; because they are tired, the clients leg is heavy and hard to maneuver, or they just do not like to massage people.

Procedure

1. Let the cream warm before you begin, by placing it into the electric heater well.
2. Apply a generous amount of hand cream into both palms before touching the client's leg.
3. Begin at right below the kneecap.
4. Use slow, deep **petrissage** kneading motions in a circular motion, working from the back of the calf to the sides of the leg, and all the way down to the ankle.

5. At the ankle, using both hands in a sandwich-style embrace of the foot, cross your full hands over the front of the leg, working back up to the knee. Rotate your wrists as you work in an upward direction.
6. Repeat this movement as the hands work back down towards the ankle again.

   Although all of the above movements can be repeated several times, they should be repeated at least twice on each leg.
7. While supporting the leg with one hand, grasp the heel of the same foot and slowly rotate it clockwise.
8. Using the thumb, work small circles up the center of the sole of the foot.
9. Gently grasp each toe separately and massage the top, bottom and sides of each toe.
10. Grasp the top of the foot with both hands and gently rotate and pull the foot upward and downward. This stretches the Achilles tendon.
11. Making both hands sandwich the foot, twist and rotate the entire foot.

    All of these movements should also be repeated at least twice.

NOTE

Many manicurists allow the client's other foot to remain soaking while the other foot is being massaged. It does allow the foot to stay warm, however, it also waterlogs the skin. The toes may look shriveled and prune-like. It would be better to wrap the other foot in a heated bootie, or pre-warmed towel.

The same steps are repeated on the other leg and foot. As the second leg is being massaged, the finished foot is slipped into a heated bootie or preheated towel.

Although it does vary with each manicurist, the standard amount of time to massage BOTH legs and feet is generally under ten minutes.

The hand cream is used more for slippage during massage than chosen for its revitalizing capabilities. Often the excess is just wiped off. If a polish is scheduled, alcohol is used to remove the cream from the nails so that the polish will stick properly. Toe separators are then put in place and the nails are painted with base coat, color, and top coat. This completes the standard pedicure.

Creating the Perfect Aromatherapy Pedicure

Nail salons that decide to go the extra mile to offer the aromatherapy pedicure, are also likely to decide to invest in a whirlpool spa chair. The major differences between the standard pedicure and the aromatherapy pedicure are:

1. The customizing of the oils used in the massage.
2. The ability to create a mixture that brings about an immediate change in the appearance of the skin.
3. The attention to the client's skin is equal to the time spent on the nails.

Aromatherapy Pedicure Equipment and Supplies

One pedicure table

One light/lamp source

One heater for oils or creams (a baby bottle warmer works well)

Individual plastic liners for the heater

Cotton

Brand new orangewood sticks

Brand new nail file

Sterilized foot baths (one for cleaning, one for rinsing); OR standard plastic foot bath with electric heater and vibrating motor; OR spa chair (with whirlpool jets and vibrating massage motors)

Sterilized nail clippers

Sterilized cuticle scissors

Sterilized nail brush

Roll of paper towels

Full selection of nail polishes

Alcohol (Rubbing or 70% isopropyl alcohol)

Nail polish remover

Cuticle remover lotion/cream

Separate trolley (to hold all the essential oils, beakers, baby bottle warmer)

Electric booties

Crock-Pot (crockery cooking pot) for warming dry towels

Essential oils

CAUTION

It is very important to make sure that the oils are hydrosoluble for the whirlpool pipes and drains. Some essential oils build up and clog the pipes/drains of this very expensive bath. Be sure to check with the supplier to determine the correct composition. Most companies offer both kinds of oils.

Pre-Massage Procedure

As in the standard pedicure, the client is instructed to come into the salon with the open-toed shoes, and loose-fitting pants. The polish is selected, and the client is seated in the chair, where two whirlpool jets and lumbar massager are set into action. The client soaks for 20 minutes in water that has been prepared with aromatherapy formulas with antibacterial and/or antiviral properties.

CAUTION

Special care must be practiced when using specific oils.

Remember: Rosemary, sage, eucalyptus, hyssop, fennel, and tagetes (among others) are **very dangerous** to pregnant women.

Eucalyptus and lemongrass **cannot** be used on young children.

Bergamot is **very dangerous** to any client with photosensitivity.

Aromatherapy Antibacterial and Antiviral Formulations

Antibacterial

Formula #1: Mix 25 drops eucalyptus, 15 drops onion and 25 drops tea tree into the bath water.

Antiviral

Formula #1: Mix 30 drops thyme, 30 drops tagetes, and 20 drops eucalyptus lemon into the bath water. If the water jets of the foot bath do not mix the oils, add a touch of alcohol to get them to blend. Remember, essential oils are lipophilic, and therefore do not mix well with just water.

For Pregnant Women

Antibacterial formula: Add to bath water: 15 drops clove, 30 drops tea tree and 10 drops lavender.

Antiviral formula: Add to bath water: 30 drops tagetes, 40 drops sandalwood, and 10 drops oregano.

CAUTION

As always check for allergies and sensitivities before making a blend.

A partial list of essential oils known to have **antibacterial properties** includes: balsam de Peru, bergamot, chamomile, cinnamon, clove, eucalyptus, eucalyptus lemon, eucalyptus radiata, garlic, hyssop, lavender, lemon oil, lime, myrtle, nerouli, nutmeg, onion, oregano, patchouli, pine, ravensara, sarriette, tea tree, terebinth, and thyme.

Essential oils with **antiviral properties** include: cinnamon, clove, eucalyptus lemon, eucalyptus radiata, garlic, lavender, onion, oregano, ravensara, sandalwood, tea tree, and thyme.

Aromatherapy Pedicure Massage

The area that an aromatherapy pedicure excels in is in the massage. All the movements can be the same as described in the standard pedicure massage (page 162). Custom-designing the oils to fit each client separately is the distinguishable, and invaluable part. The skin on clients' legs and feet will change from the very first application. Unlike the standard hand cream, which is filled with wax and fillers, the essential oils are pure. They will melt into the skin with ease and be completely absorbed.

Aromatherapy Formulas that Replace Standard (Massage) Hand Cream

For Dry Skin

Formula #1: Warm 2 oz. apricot kernel oil and add: 5 drops geranium. Stir and it is ready to use.

This formula will leave the skin smooth and generating a light fragrance. The client will find this refreshing.

Formula #2: Warm 2 oz. hazelnut oil and add: 3 drops jasmine, 3 drops neroli, and 3 drops carrot. Stir and it is ready to use.

The aroma will give the client the aromatic sensation of being transformed to the Orient. This formula will leave the skin satiny.

Formula #3: Warm 2 oz. jojoba oil and add: 4 drops chamomile and 4 drops patchouli. Stir.

For sensitive skinned clients. This formula will solve the dryness problem without leaving the skin feeling any residue.

Formula #4: Warm 2 oz. sesame oil and add: 5 drops sandalwood. Stir.

This formula is not gender-specific, however most men with dry skin will like this formula best. It has a woodsy fragrance.

Key essential oils for **dry skin** include: benzoin, carrot, chamomile, geranium, hyssop, neroli, patchouli, palmarosa, rose, and sandalwood.

For Oily Skin

Formula #1: Begin with 2 oz. soya bean oil and add: 5 drops lemon. Stir and it is ready to use.

This formula will leave the skin feeling refreshed. Perfect for oily skin, since it leaves almost no residue.

Formula #2: Begin with 2 oz. borage seed oil and add: 3 drops lavender, 3 drops rosemary, and 3 drops thyme. Stir.

The thyme will leave the skin tingly and the lavender will offer a light oriental essence.

Formula #3: Begin with 2 oz. grapeseed oil and add: 4 drops petitgrain and 4 drops violet leaf oil. Stir.

This formulation is very light in fragrance, which will be perfect for those clients who prefer not to have a heavy lingering scent.

Formula #4: Begin with 2 oz. evening primrose oil and add: 5 drops thyme.

This formula will tingle. The sensation will be somewhat like a cool heat. Men will especially like this formulation.

Key essential oils for **oily skin** include: bergamot, eucalyptus, juniper, lavender, lemon oil, palmarosa, patchouli, peppermint, petitgrain, rosemary, sandalwood, thyme, and violet leaf oil.

Chapter 12

Aromatherapy Massage

Aromatherapy massage has been around for centuries in other parts of the world. Historians have documented the Romans and Greeks used aromatherapy massage as part of their royal rituals. In the United States, it has become the current trend. Aromatherapy massage may not have a long history of use in America, but it is here to stay. It is worth mentioning that aromatherapy massage is fast becoming the chosen style for "in-home" sessions, too. Thousands of couples across the country, are incorporating aromatherapy oils into their private backrubs. Their children's children will know of it as the chosen way to get a massage.

Functions of Aromatherapy Massage

Aromatherapy massage can be done as a spot treatment. In fact, it is most often incorporated as part of a facial, where the aromatherapy massage is used only on the face, ears, neck, shoulders and décolleté (deep neckline) area. It is used in manicures and pedicures for the hands, fingers, wrists, forearms and feet. It is used as part of the head massage for hairdressers for the scalp, nape and hair.

Aromatherapy massage is most appreciated when it is done for the whole body. Aromatherapy massage simply takes all the stresses and strains out of the body. It works from the outside to the inside of the brain.

CAUTION

In dealing with all skin tissue, the chance for an allergic reaction is very much a concern. Also remember that the client's air passages are connected to their eyes, ears and throat. Breathing the essences of a known allergen can bring about serious and severe reactions

---

Criteria for Performing Massages

Besides needing to know if the client has any known allergies, there are other medical conditions that are important to know exist. These could make you decide to postpone the session or even refuse the service all together. The cliche "When in doubt, don't" fits here. Following are just a few of the major important ones to consider.

- If the client is undergoing any chemotherapy, they cannot receive a massage.
- If the client has epilepsy, or is prone to any other type of seizure, a massage is not in order without a doctor's written approval.
- If the client is under care for high blood pressure, or has any heart malady of any kind, massage is prohibited.
- If the client is a diabetic, get written consent from the doctor before proceeding with the massage.
- If the client is pregnant, the treatment will have to change to accommodate this. Get written consent from her OB/GYN before proceeding with any treatment.
- If the client has any form of rash or dermatitis (visible skin irritation), do not proceed with a massage.
- If the client has full-body acne, forego any massage. There is a strong risk of spreading the infection through the whole system, and getting the bacteria trapped under the masseuse/masseur's fingernails.
- If the client has any fungus under the fingernails or toenails, it is advisable not to do the massage until they seek medical assistance and get it cleared up. It is advisable to avoid those areas, and perform the massage on the rest of the body. Remember the cliche: "when in doubt, don't."

If the state in which you live requires you to have a massage license before you can perform a massage on the public, then the same licensure requirement holds true for an aromatherapy massage. Both the standard massage and an aromatherapy massage require partial or complete nudity for the client, direct skin contact between you and the client, and a product to be used for slippage.

Many states require that you provide a shower for the client to use after the service is rendered. The current trend is to have the client shower at home before the massage. Here are some of the reasons why:

- It benefits both the masseuse/masseur and the client.
- The masseuse/masseur does not have to deal with unnecessary body odors.
- The client's skin will actual benefit from the warmth and moisture the shower provides.
- It complies with the law, while keeping the masseuse/masseur on a better schedule. The shower time is before the treatment, therefore, no one is a last minute no-show.
- The essential oils penetrate so completely that the need for subsequent rinsing is not usually necessary.

With an aromatherapy massage, the essential oils penetrate even more effectively on clean, warm, moist skin. In the more traditional standard Swedish massage, the oils selected are usually thick and leave a significant film all over the surface of the body. Because this thick oil was the standard massage vehicle for decades, a shower after the session was required by state statute.

Characteristics of Aromatherapy Massage

There are some similarities between an aromatherapy massage and a standard Swedish massage. Both follow all the typical movements that deal with the muscles of the body. Both can use ointments and/or slippage materials. Aromatherapy is closely linked to holistic health practices. Shiatsu and acupressure are holistic massages. These two concepts are considered "dry" treatments, meaning no oil of any kind is used. Therefore, aromatherapy essential oils are not compatible with them.

Choosing Essential Oils for Massage

Essential oils are known to have properties that can affect all the organs inside our bodies. Refer to the "Quick Reference Guide to Essential Oils" (Chapter 3, pages 18 to 28) for the complete background of each of the most commonly used essential oils. The base/carrier oil will be one of the 17 chosen from the list on page 28.

For an aromatherapy massage, the professional should have at least the following 25 essential oils to choose from:

1. Benzoin	14. Lemon
2. Bois de rose	15. Marjoram
3. Carrot	16. Neroli
4. Chamomile	17. Orange
5. Clary sage	18. Palmarosa
6. Cypress	19. Patchouli
7. Fennel	20. Peppermint
8. Frankincense	21. Petitgrain
9. Geranium	22. Rose
10. Hyssop	23. Rosemary
11. Jasmine	24. Sandalwood
12. Juniper	25. Ylang-ylang
13. Lavender	

At least four ounces of product is needed for a full body aromatherapy massage. The basic formula consists of 4 ounces of one of the base oils and then an additional 10–15 drops of the essential oil(s). The solution is best received by the skin if it is gently warmed. A baby bottle warmer works best. Keep the beaker inside the warmer for the duration of the massage. This will keep it at a constant warm temperature. You can also run the sides of the beaker under very warm/hot water or put it in a microwave oven for under 5 seconds. These last two methods will not keep the oil warm for the duration of the massage.

Whether selecting the standard Swedish massage or customizing the treatment with an aromatherapy massage, the most popular service is a one-hour full-body massage. This gives the client a wonderful experience without the masseuse/masseur becoming too tired doing it. Stamina is an important factor when booking the sessions.

NOTE

It is necessary that you keep up on proper personal exercise. You will need upper body strength to keep a full day's worth of appointments.

Creating the Proper Atmosphere

It is important to set up the massage room to be very comfortable for the client's personal needs. The lights should be very dim. The room must be spotless, with clean sheets, towels, and dressing gowns for each client. This will make a lot of laundry! The floor should be carpeted or have a large rug on it. This keeps down the noise from the masseuse/masseur walking around the room. It also acts like an insulator of outside noises. Most places are not made to be sound-proofed when they are first constructed.

Soft music is highly recommended. Some practitioners use tapes with subliminal messages, some with nature sounds like ocean waves or rain forests. The clients choose which they want to hear. The tapes should be one hour long. If not, use a tape player with auto-reverse on it. You **should not** stop the massage to turn the tape over.

Having a heat lamp allows the client to feel warm during the entire massage. Be careful to make sure it is not positioned too close to the skin. The client may think it feels great, only to get a mild burn after the hour is up. Some rooms are too small to have the lamp conveniently placed on the floor and still have enough walking room to move about freely. If you find yourself in this situation, the following alternative is one solution (gained from personal experience) to give you enough room and keep the customer comfortable. The old adage "necessity is the mother of invention" applies here. Here is what to do if placed in a room too tiny to comfortably fit the table, heat lamp and yourself:

1. Take a sheet (that may normally be draped in half) and completely open it over the table. Both sides will fall to the floor on either side of the table.
2. The client will come in and lie down, using one towel to cover the breasts (for females), and one towel to cover the genitals.
3. When the client is ready, you enter and take both sides of the sheet and bring the edges over the client, so they meet in the middle. Now the client is covered like a loosely fitted cocoon.
4. As you work on an area, peel the sheet back, leaving the rest of the body covered. This keeps them from getting cold. (In fact, it has an additional value not first considered when devising this system: it offers a feeling of modesty, which is greatly appreciated by everyone.)

I received so many compliments on this approach, that I now use this cocoon method, no matter where I work, in rooms large and small, with or without heat lamps.

Another added piece of equipment is needed to hold and/or prepare heated towels. A hot towel caddy is wonderful to have, but the cheaper way to go is to use a Crock-Pot (a crockery cooking pot). Keep it on the lowest setting. It is most common to use four towels per massage: two for the back, and one for each foot. At the end of the massage, it is easy to wipe down the entire body to remove the tiny thin film that may be left. Often after the hot towel is used, the client does not feel that a shower is even needed. Not showering allows the essential oils a longer time to do their special "magic," after the session is over.

Standard Massage Movements

Aromatherapy massage can be performed using any method of hand movement. All of the standard finger positions of the Swedish massage will do just nicely with this treatment.

Effleurage

The first and most popular massage movement is **effleurage.** Effleurage uses the flat portion of the palms and fingers to exert even pressure on all the parts of your hand. Use full strokes with your hands. The movements can be short or long. The pressure can be gentle or firm. You have complete freedom to adjust your movements to suit each client's personal preference.

Effleurage is a very flexible movement. It can encompass large areas like the back or legs, or be used on the cheeks of the face. When doing a full body massage, the masseuse/masseur must be able to pace themselves so as to complete the treatment with the same amount of energy. Effleurage does not require a high degree of energy. In fact, the masseuse/masseur can use their own body weight to help maintain the energy level while using effleurage motions.

Effleurage movements have wonderful stress-reducing effects on the body from the inside out, including:

- Relaxation of any muscle group is assured.
- All the nerve endings are calmed and soothed.
- The blood flow rebalances and circulation increases to all of the extremities.
- Overall tensions are minimized.

Petrissage

There are other movements to the standard massage that fit perfectly in an aromatherapy massage. **Petrissage** is one of these. If you can imagine the motion of your hands when you knead a mound of

dough, like making bread, then you have a good idea how this movement works. You have to decide where to use this action. Areas that
are especially receptive are the fat-collecting parts, like the stomach,
thighs and backs. The movements should not look like you are at-
tacking the body, but rather be slow and carefully planned. You want
to move the skin, but not cause uncomfortable sensations, or pain.
You also do not want to cause the area to bruise hours after the massage is over.

Petrissage, done properly, will increase circulation deep into the
muscles, fat deposits, and skin tissue. This offers total relaxation for
overworked muscles. It also aids the flow of lymphatic fluid within
the lymph system. It is worth noting this is *not part of lymphatic
drainage techniques*. Petrissage has a secondary effect on the lymph,
not a direct one. It does directly effect the release of toxins from the
fatty deposit areas. With the increase in circulation, the lymph system can then take the toxins away from the area.

For beginners, it is easy to use too strong thumb pressure when
performing the kneading action. Use light thumb pressure until you
have improved your technique to where all five fingers are exerting
even amounts of pressure in unison. For practice, the masseuse/
masseur can use their own knee cap for pressure sensitivity, and the
top of their own thighs for unison movement of both hands.

Tapotement

Tapotement is another movement that can be used on the face,
especially around the eyes and mouth. Some people call this the
"piano" motion, because it follows the action the fingers would take
over piano keys. The trick to master tapotement is to have even tapping movement for each finger. Most people have strong index
(pointer) fingers, and weaker end and pinky fingers. Practicing on piano keys is an excellent way to gain dexterity in all of your fingers on
both hands. If a piano is not available, you can roll a thick towel and
wet it. As you move your fingers over the towel, you will see what in-
dentations are being made. You want these to be the same.

Chopping

There is another motion that works well on the back of the shoulder
blades and the back of the legs. Many call it the **"chop"** or chopping. To chop, use the outer edge of both hands rotating up and
down over the area. This is a very vigorous movement, and not for
the timid. Clients who have very strong, hard bodies, love to have

this performed all over their torsos and full legs. It takes quite a lot of
energy and force to do it properly. You will want to do this when you
are fresh and full of pep, as it can drain your own energy fairly quickly.

> **NOTE**
> Every masseuse/masseur will determine what works best
> for their own personal comfort. Stamina comes with ex-
> perience and working out. You will have to decide how
> many massages you can do one after the other. I live in
> California, where there is no distinction between male
> and female workers or patrons. I am short and will never
> have tremendous upper body strength. Therefore, I work
> one male massage session to every three female sessions,
> and will never last longer than four full body treatments
> in a row. I usually take breaks for 5–7 minutes between
> appointments. You will find the right limit for yourself.

Beginning and Performing Massage

Where to start the massage can vary with each individual and preference. There is no "one way" to do it. Most often the massage begins
with the client lying on his or her back. Start the massage at the top
of their heads and work to the feet, but **always move the blood
towards the heart.** Then have them turn over and work from the
feet towards the head. This gives a full 360-degree circle, encompass-
ing all 2,000 meridian points and all seven chakras (pronounced
shah-crahs).

In yoga philosophy **meridian points** are where strong nerve
cells control various other nerve cells in the surrounding tissue. In
layman's terms, meridians are like supervisors to a very large team of
coworkers. Removing the stress stored in the meridian has a direct effect on removing all stress within its territory. It would be virtually
impossible to individually drain all the stress from millions of nerve
cells within the whole body. By manually working the 2,000 points,
you reach all of them.

In shiatsu and acupressure, the meridian points have to be
worked in a synchronized manner to bring about balance and harmony within the body. This is not so when using standard massage
movements. While your hands manipulate the various muscles and
skin, you automatically touch various meridians. Also, according to

yoga philosophy, chakras are the color and/or energy fields sur-rounding the body. Each controls a specific physical and mental health area. They begin at the head and wind down to the very top of the thighs. These fields are not visible to the eye. They are not painful. There are many that do not believe in things that are not tangible. People decide for themselves what they want to believe. Re-gardless, an aromatherapy massage will only enhance the chakra fields.

Your "Signature" Style

With time and practice you should eventually be able to create your own "signature" style of massage. The use of essential oils will not be the only "key" for your "signature," because the client's body will be the major determinate for which essential oils will be selected.

Massaging Specific Areas

Please do not take the following ideas as the only way to perform a full body massage, although certainly, beginners may want to start with them.

The Abdomen

Effleurage is the key movement of choice for massaging abdomens. Use the flat part of all of your fingers, but not your palms. Begin the movement on the client's LEFT side. Following a CLOCKWISE mo-tion three times, making full circles across the stomach. Then reverse to the COUNTERCLOCKWISE motion three times. Many people are ticklish on their stomachs. Using a slow, firm pressure, should avoid sending them into giggles. For people who have extending skin in their tummies, adjust your movements to those described in the next section. Otherwise, you may just have the sensation that the client has "swallowed" your hands, as they appear to sink inside of the loose skin. Clients who are overweight, or females who have had many children, can have this problem.

Abdomens with Excessive, Stretched Skin

Gently but firmly place your nondominant hand and forearm across the center of the client's stomach. Do the above-mentioned movements for abdomens on the LEFT side first. Then repeat on the other side. Do not remove the stationary hand and forearm until the massage for this area is complete. This will make the movements easy, and the client's stomach will not jiggle and shake. The clients will appreciate this, and be less self-conscious about their bodies.

The Arms

Petrissage is the chosen movement for arm massage. Knead the muscles on the forearm and the biceps of the upper arm. You can do it with one hand or two. Many practitioners usually support the client's arm with one hand and massage with the other.

The Back

The chopping, effleurage, or petrissage can be the chosen movements to massage the back. Using a combination of all three is very helpful in keeping your fingers and hands from tiring too quickly. It is usually appreciated to have a firm pressure in all of the movements.

> ### CAUTION
> The only area that you do not work is the actual vertebrae. Manipulation of the vertebrae should be left to chiropractors.

If you choose to start with effleurage, begin at the lower back (lumbar region), using both hands. Work up the back, going over the top of the shoulders and back down the sides of the back. Repeat this action at least five times, then stop at the shoulder blade and perform several rotations of the chop. Follow this action with the kneading of petrissage on the sides of the back. Almost everyone loves to have their backs massaged. It is one part of the body that you can never work on for too long.

The Face

Effleurage, petrissage and tapotement are all used to massage facial muscles and skin. It will be necessary for you to master the sense of pressure being exerted on each and every finger. Most people find that their dominant hand powers the massage. On the face, this becomes uncomfortable for the client. The masseuse/masseur can do exercises to get both hands more evenly balanced, for pressure. During a full body massage, the beginning point is usually the forehead, moving to the temples, around the eyes, down the nose, cheeks, mouth, chin, and jaw line. The ears and neck are done at this time too.

Shiatsu pressure points are easily accessed during this massage. Although it is not necessary to worry about getting all the points pressurized, there are several that are high stress collectors and, thus, need to be addressed. These are the pressure points around the eyes, temples, and sinus areas. Placing the thumbs on each side of the bridge of the nose, and spread the rest of the finger pads around the area directly under the eye sockets. Pulse the finger pads three times. Slide the fingertips to the sides of the temples and perform the same three pressure pulses.

To release the stress out of the jaw and cheek, use the flat side of the fingers and effleurage rotation movements. Roll over the jaw and fleshy part of the cheeks, alternating hands. It works well to get a rhythm going, eliminating the chance to create a slapping sensation with the dominant hand.

Next, place index and middle fingers along the sides of the client's mouth. At the same time place the ring and pinky finger on the top and bottom of the chin. Press three times and release as the fingers glide along the entire jaw bone. Work toward the temple, press there three times. Repeat this movement at least three times.

Using the full fingers to slide/glide over the entire forehead area, smoothe out the large frontalis muscle. So many clients crinkle up their foreheads and the muscle gets set into deep ridges.

Using petrissage kneading movements, over the zygomatic (major and minor) muscles, helps restore tone and increase the circulation to these powerful controllers of expression. Women are particularly sensitive to the zygomatics (cheek areas) folding and losing their firmness. Manipulating these muscles through massage, is similar to aerobic exercising of the body. Increased tone and strength can be accomplished with repeat treatments.

Tapotement's "piano" movements should be done over the eyes and mouth. The obicularis oculi, and obicularis oris are circular muscles that respond well to this massage technique. At first, it takes strong concentration to get all four fingers moving evenly and in harmony with each other (remember the rolled wet towel exercise.)

The Feet

Effleurage is for comforting, and petrissage for detoxing the feet. (REFLEXOLOGY is a holistic foot massage that falls into its own special category.) Begin with the toes and work to the heel. You will use your thumbs more than any other finger. Feet are the most ticklish area of the body due to the thousands of nerve cells on the bottoms of the feet. Firm pressure is the key to a good foot massage.

Wrapping the feet in warm towels will make it a better treatment. If there are thick calluses on the client's feet, suggest a pedicure. If the client's feet show signs of fungus or rashes, and you did not detect it before you started the massage, there is something you can do. Keep a pair of latex gloves in your lab coat. Quickly slip them on, and continue the massage, avoiding all areas that the fungus has affected.

The Legs

Effleurage, petrissage and chopping can all be used to massage the legs. Begin with upward motions, starting at the ankles and working towards the thighs. Effleurage will calm the legs if they are tired. Use your fingers and palms together. Petrissage kneading will help detoxify the thigh areas, particularly if they have cellulite. Your thumbs will be the major force in this action. Chopping works well on cellulite, too.

The Neck

Effleurage is the chosen massage movement for the neck. Gentle, firm, circular action is best. Start at the base of the neck and work toward the base of the occipital bone. Again, remember **NOT** to put pressure on the vertebrae. Repeat this movement four times. The neck is the second favorite area to be massaged.

CAUTION

Do not put pressure on the vertebrae when massaging the neck or back.

The Shoulders

Effleurage and petrissage are the chosen massage movements for shoulders. A lot of people hold their stress in their shoulders. Knead the muscles from the outer edges into the center. Both hands are used, with your thumbs and palms being the strong force in your actions. On a large client, or one that is especially muscular, this will take a large degree of your strength. Your stamina will determine how long you can keep massaging the shoulders.

> **NOTE**
>
> When you begin your aromatherapy massage **on any area of the body,** place your hands firmly on the client. Ask if the pressure you are using feels "just right", or if they would appreciate a milder or heavier pressure. Never start the question with a negative remark: "Is this too hard, or rough?" The client may not have any idea how the pressure should be, and asking the question in a negative statement only begins the session with doubt. Remember positive energy yields positive results, and negative energy yields negative results.

Preparing the "Holistic You"

Since aromatherapy and holistic health run very close together, it may be noteworthy to offer you some guidelines that have been used for decades when offering clients various holistic services.

Aromatherapy is just one part of the holistic concept. Remember that a major characteristic of the holistic concept is positive energy fields. It would be unrealistic to think that you can walk into work, with a natural smile on your lips and a twinkle in your eyes every single day of your life. Life can be challenging for all of us. The conflict arises when your clients are expecting you to be "up, positive, and happy-go-lucky" each and every time they have an appointment to see you. It is part of why they come to you in the first place. They want to be made to feel better, and you are there to wait on them to make that happen. So on particularly challenging days, here is what can help get you through it:

- Count to ten backwards before you walk through the door. When you reach 1, exhale all of your oxygen, inhale deeply and smile.
- If your fingers are cold (and when you are under stress, they usually are), run them under very warm water, or hold a hot towel with both hands to get them warmed up.
- If you still feel a bit negative, vigorously shake your hands, before starting the massage.
- Before you perform the service, remove your shoes. Energy transfer occurs between you and the client. If the client is full of stress and tension, it enters you through your fingertips, and leaves through your toes. In fact, wearing 100% white

cotton socks is also helpful. The socks absorb part of the toxins that your feet fill up with during the treatment.

- If you suffer from odorous feet, wear a clean pair for each massage to eliminate the problem. Otherwise, sprinkling a half corn starch and half talc mixture inside of your socks will help.

These steps may seem odd to you at first, but they do work. Living your life in a more holistic consciousness, will become a major asset in all aspects of your life. Being able to offer a more positive, uplifting atmosphere at work will make your boss, fellow coworkers, and your clients very happy.

Aromatherapy Body Massage Oil Formulas

With all of these formulas, you begin with a baby bottle warmer and a 120 mL sterile glass beaker. Fill the beaker with 1–1 ½ inches of water, and bring it to a boil or soft simmer. Place a plastic container inside of this hot water, to heat the oils inside. The reason you do not use the glass beaker to hold the oils, is that during the session your hands will be oily and grabbing a glass beaker is an accident waiting to happen. This way the heated water keeps the plastic container warm but not melted. The oil stays warm, but not too hot, and you can lift the plastic container in and out as you need the oil without the fear of shattering glass everywhere. (If this sounds like it was learned from experience . . . it was!)

Keeping the oil formulas warm, but not boiling, throughout the session provides a more enjoyable experience for the client, and it keeps the masseuse/masseur's hands from getting as tired. The warmth of the oil helps keep the joints in the fingers more agile.

CAUTION

Special care must be practiced when using specific oils.

Remember: Rosemary, sage, eucalyptus, hyssop, fennel, and tagetes (among others) are **very dangerous** to pregnant women.

Eucalyptus and lemongrass **cannot** be used on young children.

Bergamot is **very dangerous** to any client with photosensitivity.

For Dry Skin

Formula #1: Warm 4 oz. apricot kernel oil and add: 15 drops geranium. Stir and it is ready to use.

This formula will leave the skin smooth with a light, lingering fragrance. The client will find this refreshing.

Formula #2: Warm 4 oz. hazelnut oil and add: 5 drops jasmine, 5 drops neroli, and 5 drops carrot. Stir, and it is ready.

The client will have the aromatic sensation of being transformed to the Orient. This formula will leave the skin satiny.

Formula #3: Warm 4 oz. jojoba oil and add: 7 drops chamomile and 8 drops patchouli. Stir.

For sensitive skinned clients, this formula will solve the dryness problem without leaving residue for the skin to feel.

Formula #4: Warm 4 oz. sesame oil and add: 15 drops sandalwood. Stir.

This formula knows no gender, however most men with dry skin will like this formula best. It has a woodsy fragrance.

Key essential oils for dry skin are: Benzoin, carrot, chamomile, geranium, hyssop (use sparingly), neroli, patchouli, palmarosa, rose, and sandalwood.

For Oily Skin

Formula #1: Begin with 4 oz. soya bean oil and add: 15 drops lemon oil. Stir. It is ready to use.

This formula will leave the skin refreshed. Perfect for oily skin, since it leaves almost no residue.

Formula #2: Begin with 4 oz. borage seed oil and add: 10 drops lavender, 3 drops rosemary, and 2 drops thyme. Stir.

The thyme will leave the skin tingly, and the lavender will offer a light, oriental sensation.

Formula #3: Begin with 4 oz. grapeseed oil and add: 7 drops petitgrain, and 8 drops violet leaf oil. Stir.

This formulation is very light in fragrance, which will be perfect for those clients who prefer not to have a heavy, lingering scent.

Formula #4: Begin with 4 oz. evening primrose oil and add: 15 drops thyme.

This formula will tingle. The sensation will be somewhat like cool heat. Men will especially like this formulation.

Key essential oils for oily skin are: Bergamot, eucalyptus, juniper, lavender, lemon oil, palmarosa, patchouli, peppermint, petitgrain, rosemary, sandalwood, thyme, and violet leaf oil.

Special Tips and Tricks for the Client Who is "Allergic to Everything"

As a professional, you will encounter clients who are allergic to almost everything. What do you do? Obviously you can turn them away, but who really benefits from that decision? It is a proven fact that IF YOU CAN EAT IT, YOU CAN HAVE IT PUT ON YOUR SKIN!

Here are just some of the possibilities:

Use regular cooking oil for the base. Vegetable, canola, corn oil, are just a few of the many available oils. Then, instead of mixing essential oils with the base, use pure extracts from the spice section of any grocery store. Pure vanilla, pure ginger, pure cinnamon, pure orange, pure lemon, and or pure peach extracts are just a few to choose from.

The vanilla is great for calming. Ginger and cinnamon work for invigorating the skin. Orange extract works well for smokers. Peach is excellent for dry skin. The same 15-drop formulation as described in formulas 1–4 above is ok to use for these selections.

Part 3

Appendices

Appendix A

Suppliers of Aromatherapy Oils and Equipment

The following is a list of companies that specialize in serving the professional cosmetology and/or aromatherapy customer. They will sell products that can be retailed in the salon. A brief description of the products/services follows each vendor entry.

Aroma Vera
Culver City, California 90231
800–669–9514
Seventy essential oils. Diffusers and various hair and skin care products. Private label products available, too.

Australian School of Awareness
251 Dorset Road
Croydon
Victoria 3136
Attn: Margaret Tozer
011–03–723–2531
FAX 011–059–646404
Privately made essential oils.

The Bayou Blending Company
210 Leonpacher Road
Lafayette, Louisiana 70508
318–234–5804 FAX 318–234–5706
Specializes in custom making any of the essential oils. Small orders are acceptable.

Essentially Yours, Ltd. (England)
366–368 London Road
Westcliff on Sea, Essex SSO 7H2 UK
011–0702–390625
Full line of essential oils and diffusers.

Essentially Yours Canada
254 Hart Street
Coquitlam B.C. CANADA V3K4A6
Full line of essential oils and diffusers.

Essentially Yours North America
PO Box 81866
Bakersfield, California 93380
Full line of essential oils and diffusers.

European College of Natural Therapies
16 North Parade
Belfast
BT7 2GG
Attn: Mary Thompson
011–0232–641454

Judith Jackson Aromatherapy
10 Serenity Lane
Cos Cob, Connecticut 06807
203–661–0295 FAX 203–622–6320
Aromatherapy products for skin care.

Ledet Oils
4611 Awani Ct.
Fair Oaks, California 95628
916–965–7546
Full line of essential oils and massage oils.

Legion of Light Productions
PO Box 1557
Mount Shasta, California 96067
Attn: Neil Cohen or Taryn Riffey
916–938–1461
Various aromatherapy products

Original Swiss Aromatics
PO Box 606
San Rafael, California 94915
415–459–3998
Full line of essential oils.

Shirley Price Aromatherapy Ltd.
Essentia House
Upper Bond Street
Hinckley
Leics
LE10 1RS
011–0455–615466
FAX 011–0455–615054
Company made essential oils.

Source Vital
3637 West Alabama
Suite 240
Houston, Texas 77027
800-880-6457
Natural organic aromatherapy products

Essential oils can also be purchased at most health food stores. Their prices will be competitive, but these products will not be able to be retailed in the salon. One of the key advantages to using health food stores as a supplier of essential oils, is that no minimum orders (i.e.: 10 bottles/cases per purchase or certain monetary amount) are required when purchasing.

Appendix B

Quick Reference to the Most Commonly Used Essential Oils

BASIL   (top note) USE WITH CARE. Although this herb is used in many food recipes, do NOT confuse it with being gentle, as an aromatherapy oil.

Primary use: To unclog congested, sluggish skin. Works as a natural insect repellent.

BENZOIN   (base note) "Friar Balsam" is a common nickname for this essential oil.

Primary use: To regenerate mature, inelastic skin. It helps to moisturize dry skin. Also good for chapped, dry and cracked hands. As in all base notes, it is warm and sedating to the skin. The clients should enjoy this essential oil as it is being massaged on them.

BERGAMOT   (top note) **CAUTION:** Extra care must be used, because the oil makes the skin photosensitive. Bergamot is never to be used directly or full strength upon the skin. It is strongly suggested that the clients wear sunscreens on areas bergamot is to be used.

Primary use: For all oily skin and hair, and seborrhea of the scalp. Acne conditions and rosacea also respond well to it. IF you know that the client is an active outdoors person and will NOT use sun protection, choose another essential oil for your formula. The professional who uses this essential oil as part of their treatment, MUST ALSO PROTECT THEIR OWN HANDS WITH A SUNSCREEN.

CAMPHOR   (middle note) **CAUTION:** It must not be used during pregnancy. Very small amounts should be used. The Golden Rule particularly applies to this essential oil. Where 4–5 drops of other oils would be fine, 1–3 drops will do nicely for this one.

Primary use: For oily skin and hair. If used, is generally included in products that are washed off; such as cleansers, shampoos, and masks rather than moisturizers.

CARROT   (middle note) This essential oil has the power to stain the skin, nails, and scalp. Care must be taken not to use it "neat" (straight on the skin).

Primary use: For all skin, hair, and nail care that needs revitalizing and moisturizing. It also has a calming effect on the skin and cuticles.

CEDARWOOD   (base note) With its natural woodsy aroma, this essential oil will appeal to men and anyone else who enjoys the smell of the outdoors. However, clients that have allergies to wood spurs and other forest elements, will not do well with this essential oil.

Primary use: Hair care: this essential oil is helpful in treating alopecia, dandruff, and seborrhea of the scalp. Skin care: for oily skin and irritations.

CHAMOMILE GERMAN   (middle note) It is particularly mild and gentle and can be used on young children. The practitioner will find that this essential oil has broad appeal for its natural aroma and versatile usage.

Primary use: For all skin and nails that are sensitive, dry, or irritated. With nails, if they are cracked and chapped, this essential oil is very effective. Use on scalps that are dry or flaky. Capillary distention such as couperose, is helped. It will also soothe acne and eczema.

CHAMOMILE ROMAN   (middle note) Used similarly to chamomile German, above. It also shares its treatment selection variety and broad appeal.

CINNAMON   (top note) A very potent essential oil. USE VERY SPARINGLY. Too much in skin potions can cause irritations. Not to be used "neat," or unadulterated. It performs well in blends where it is just a small part of the formula.

Primary use: Skin and nail care: It works very well to tone the skin, and as an antiviral in skin and nails.

CLARY SAGE   (top note) This herb is a winner with all aromatherapists. It works very quickly on the body, in many different applications. It does not have a strong positive or negative response to its aroma. It is not a scent that is widely recognized upon first contact.

Primary use: On mature skin to perk up the complexion, as a cell regenerator. It soothes any skin or nails that are inflamed. Stimulates hair growth and helps to regulate seborrhea of the scalp.

CLOVE   (top note) A very powerful and potent essential oil, so USE ONLY THE TINIEST OF DROPS. Most people are aware of it as a spice in cooking. And many will have a predetermined idea as to whether they like its natural aroma. Check with your client first, before deciding to select this as part of a blended formula.

Primary use: Helps fight bacteria in nails and skin.

CYPRESS   (middle note) Another woodsy aroma that will have a certain appeal to "outdoor lovers." But check with your client on the possibility of their having allergies to tree pollens, before selecting this oil.

Primary use: Toning the body, balancing oily skin, strengthening nails. Works as an antiseptic to all skin and nails, oxygenates broken capillaries.

EUCALYPTUS, EUCALYPTUS LEMON, EUCALYPTUS PEPPERMINT, EUCALYPTUS RADIATA   (top notes) **CAUTION:** Do NOT use on young children, or anyone with even the mildest asthmatic condition. This oil's aroma does not blend in with other essential oils' aromas. It will always dominate the blend's smell. One drop of this essential oil can equal the aroma power of 10 drops of other less aromatic selections. Once again, check with your client's preference to its smell. Many will relate its aroma to medicinal products used in their youths.

Primary use: Acne and oily skin. Great for increasing the circulation of the nail beds and cuticles. Superb scalp stimulator. An excellent antiseptic.

EVERLASTING   (top note) Similar to eucalyptus, this oil's aroma does not blend in with the aromas of other essential oils. It will always dominate the blend's smell. Once again, check with your client's preference to its smell.

Primary use: It has strong anti-inflammatory properties that are wonderful on sensitive skin, acne conditions, or any inflamed nails, cuticles, or skin. If the scalp gets inflamed after a chemical service, it will aide in reducing the redness.

FENNEL (sweet)   (middle note) **CAUTION:** Use with care, and never during pregnancy. Inside of the herb is a high phenolic ether content, thus a VERY VERY small amount is to be used in the formula. It is hard to predict your client's response to the aroma. It will go either way. Most often, the formula will only have one drop of this essential oil. The Golden Rule always fits this oil.

Primary use: For cleansers for oily skin. To revitalize mature skin and hands.

FRANKINCENSE   (base note) Not as pungent as eucalyptus, still it will dominate the blends's aroma. Check your client's preference. It will not be as recognizable as eucalyptus. Only the more advanced practitioners will find themselves turning to this essential oil a lot.

Primary use: Skincare: For calming any inflamed tissue and for toning loose skin. Nails: Excellent for treating damaged cuticles. Hair: Adds body to limp hair.

GERANIUM   (middle note) Its natural aroma has broad appeal from women of all ages. Most often men will find the aroma of this essential oil "too flowery." They might think that you are covering them in a woman's perfume.

Primary use: Multifunctional. Can be effective as a cell generator for mature skin, an astringent for oily skin, and decrease the slick found on acne skin. Offers quick repair for chapped, cracked hands and cuticles. Helps reduce the "greasy" hair sensation.

GRAPEFRUIT   (middle note) It has large universal appeal, partly due to its overwhelmingly popular aroma, and for its wide-ranging abilities.

Primary use: Uniformly used for hair, skin, and nails. No one area is stronger than the others. Hair: It reduces the slick formed by seborrhea, and reduces dandruff scales. It increases the fresh bounce to most hair. Skin: It works with toning facial and body tissue, especially tissue with cellulite. Nails: It brightens yellow nails, helps increase the oxygen flow to nails to rid buildup of residue on the nail beds. It strengthens the cuticle tissue.

HYSSOP   (middle note) **CAUTION:** Must be used with care, because it is so strong an oil. It cannot be used during pregnancy. This herb's natural aroma may not be on everyone's top ten list. Check with your client first. Very small amounts of oil are used in any formula. For most formulas, the maximum amount of drops will be two.

Primary use: For moisturizing any sensitive skin and reducing redness of couperose. Excellent for treating eczema of the scalp and skin. Will treat hands and feet for weak nails or damaged cuticles.

JASMINE   (base note) A solvent must be used to extract the oil out of the flower. Often ether is the chosen solvent. The process creates an increase in the financial pricing of the end product, the essential oil. Careful selection of the pure absolute of the jasmine flower will assure the proper oil for use. Only very small amounts of the oil are required. This flower has a strong oriental aroma, and the reaction to it will be close to 50–50 positive or negative. Clients who suffer greatly from hayfever-style allergies might not have a positive reaction to this oil.

Primary use: It has exceptional versatility. In some formulations it will reduce the oily slick off of skin and hair. While in other formulations it can be an overall moisturizer for dry skin, scalp, and nails. Due to its gentle nature, it works well with all sensitive bodies, hands and feet.

JUNIPER   (middle note) In ancient times it was the antiseptic of choice. It was considered the "rubbing alcohol" of the aromatherapy world.

Primary use: Still used as an active antiseptic for all skin and body areas, including the hands and feet. It is often part of the toning formulations for treating cellulite and flabby arms. In skin care, many acne conditions are improved and oily skin reduces its sebum levels.

LAVENDER   (middle note) Its aroma makes this essential oil very popular with all ages. It has a fine calming reaction to the internal and external parts of the body.

Primary use: This essential oil can be used on all parts of the body, even the eyes and lips. Hair: To treat alopecia and dry, brittle hair. Skin: Acne, rosacea and oily skins respond well to lavender. Most inflammation of the skin, as well as psoriasis, is reduced. On mature skin, it aids in moisture. For the hands and feet: it works beautifully to soothe and relieve chapping and cracking.

LEMON: (top note) **CAUTION:** Keep away from area directly around the eyes. It tops the list of the most favored essential oil, due to the powerful aroma of the fruit and its wide appeal with men and women alike. It would be very hard to find a person that does not like the natural fragrance of this oil.

Primary use: One of the most flexible oils of all. It can be used on every body part from the top of the scalp and hair, to the bottoms of the feet. Depending on how it is mixed, it works with oily or dry skin. It energizes the mature skin and repairs wrinkled skin to a new smoothness. For nails it clears yellowing and refreshes the nail beds and cuticles. Whether you are a beginning or an advanced practitioner, you will find that you use this essential oil often.

LEMONGRASS: (top note) **CAUTIONS:** Do not use this on chidlren. Do not use directly on the skin. Do not use on clients allergic to grass pollens. This essential oil is also known for its antiseptic properties. However, it does have the ability to act as an irritant if directly on the skin. It should not be used directly on the skin—straight, also known as "neat." In blends, use just a little bit of this essential oil. For most formulas, do not go over the four drop level.

Primary use: Predominantly used in body care, for toning, and as an antiseptic. Also used on oily or acne skin to reduce pustules—BUT only as a blend, not straight on its own.

LIME   (top note) **CAUTION:** Keep away from the eyes. A close choice to its "cousin" the lemon, its natural aroma is strongly popular with men. It is not as diversified as the lemon and not used as often.

Primary use: On the skin as an astringent and tonic.

MARJORAM   (middle note) Although it is colorless, it is also very pungent. It does not appeal to everyone. Check with your clients before selecting this essential oil for your blend.

Primary use: For treating bruising of any tissue or black-and-blue marks on the scalp, skin, hands, and feet. For damaged nail beds, such as "blackened nails," it has a positive healing quality.

MELISSA   (middle note) Clients will either find this essential oil very pleasant smelling or be repelled by its aroma. Check with the client first before making your blend.

Primary use: Nails and feet: It is a wonderful antifungal solution. Skin: Depending on the blend of the formula, acne and eczema are aided, and mature skin can be regenerated. This essential oil can be custom fit into oily or dry skin treatments.

MYRRH   (base note) A hormonal oil, this essential oil is highly recognized for its involvement in biblical history. Due to its connection, this oil has a strong aura surrounding it. Clients may respond from a deep emotional reaction to this oil, solely based on its connection to Jesus.

Primary use: Skin: Regenerates and revitalizes mature skin. For any skin that is red and sore looking, it acts as an anti-inflammatory. Nails: Reduces redness in dry, cracked hands and cuticles. Hair: Acts as an anti-inflammatory oil for scalps.

NEROLI   (top note) It has a pale yellow color. Its aroma is particularly strong and will be pleasant to many people.

Primary use: Hair: Treats scalps that are sore, or cracked and picked at. Nails: Treats bitten and torn cuticles or reddened, cracked hands and feet. Skin: Treats skin that is showing signs of irritation. This oil is perfect for tretaing sensitive skin.

NIAOULI   (top note) Its natural aura is very similar to lavender, which makes it very popular with most people.

Primary use: As a broad spectrum antiseptic solution. Skin: Improves acne and oily skin. Feet: Treats any cuts and sores.

ORANGE   (top note) It is very mild, which makes it a good choice for children and anyone with sensitive skin. Its aroma makes it one of the most popular essential oils. From the beginners to the advanced, this essential oil will be chosen often.

Primary use: Hair: It makes the hair silky smooth and shiny. Nails: It is perfect for treating rough, dry hands and feet. If the skin is weak and flabby-looking, it will revitalize it. Skin: Reduces the oil on oily and acne conditions. It helps treat congested skin. On mature skin, it improves tone and smoothness.

OREGANO   (middle note) This is a strong essential oil. It has to be used very sparingly. The aroma is so connected to food, that your clients may actually get hungry when the blend is created. It has broad appeal for both men and women.

Primary use: Body: It works very well on cellulite. Nails: It brightens the nail beds.

PALMAROSA   (middle note) This essential oil is extremely versatile. The only possible limitation will be for clients with allergies to pollens and grasses. The aroma is neither engaging nor repelling.

Primary use: Hair: It is effective in reducing limp hair. Nails: Revitalizes dry, cracked hands and nails. Also for tired feet that are dry and flaky. Skin: It energizes mature, wrinkled skin.

PARSLEY   (base note) This essential oil's appeal is based on its overall acceptance in food preparation. It helps the body clear itself of toxins.

Primary use: An effective antiseptic for skin, nails and feet. Skin: It is effective on couperose and it tones skin. Hair: It helps rid cigarette toxins from the follicles.

PATCHOULI   (base note) This oil has the ability to perform two different actions based on the quantity of the oil. Very few drops will energize, whereas many drops will relax. The exact reason is not known.

Primary use: As part of its ability to work in different reactions: it is excellent for cracked, dry hands and feet. Skin: Oily and acne skin conditions are improved and put back into balance. Hair: Restores body to oily hair.

PEPPERMINT   (top note) A very powerful essential oil, partly due to its cellular composition and partly due to its aroma. A strong favorite with young clientele. It can overwhelm the formula if its percentage of drops is significantly higher than the others. However, it can also create a popular aroma when mixed with other essential oils that have aromas that are not as pleasant.

Primary use: A major aid in reducing inflammation, irritation, and couperose. Ashy coloring of skin from smoking or prolonged sickness will brighten. On oily or acne skin, it helps reduce the congestion. Hair: It is a major tool in stimulating the scalp and loosening scales of dandruff and eczema. Nails: With its ability to oxygenate the area, it helps nails restore a healthy coloring.

PETITGRAIN   (top note) It is not as favorable in aroma to its sister oil, neroli.

Primary use: It works as a great balancer for oily conditions. Skin: Reduces oily sebum slicks and waxy buildup on acne skin. Hair: Reduces the greasy sensation on hair and scalp.

ROSE BULGAR and **ROSE MAROC**   (base notes) The potent aroma of rose oil makes it one of the most powerful and loved by women and not favored by most men. It is so gentle that it can be used on the most sensitive skins and on very young children.

Primary use: For treating all sensitive skin that is dry. On mature skin it helps reduce the signs of aging. On oily skin it reduces redness. It has a calming effect on any couperose. It soothes rough, cracked, and dry conditions on hands and feet.

ROSEMARY   (middle note) **CAUTION:** Because it naturally possesses ketones of camphor, never use it under any conditions on a pregnant woman. This essential oil will frighten the beginner, though it is not an oil that the practitioner should stay away from. Rather it is suggested that care and understanding be used. Ask questions of your supplier to assure that the oil is pure. Do not let the "purse strings" determine which oil is purchased. The best rosemary oil will be costly and worth it! It is a natural cleanser of toxins, reducer of sebum, and a cellular regenerator. This makes this essential oil one of the most diverse.

Primary use: Hair: Alopecia, dandruff, and seborrhea of the scalp all improve with use. Skin: Oily plugs and acne conditions lessen. On mature skin the cells perk up, become less wrinkled. Nails: Feet and hands will gain smoothness and increase in circulation with use.

SAGE   (top note) **CAUTION:** It SHOULD NOT BE USED ON PREGNANT WOMEN. Be careful when using sage in a blend. Its aroma may not mix well with everything.

Primary use: Hair: It is effective in reducing alopecia. Skin: It works to unclog congested skin, or improve skin that has a tendency to be sluggish.

SANDALWOOD   (base note) The woodsy aroma makes it particularly popular with men and many actively outdoor-loving women. It would be wise to check if the client has a history of allergies to grasses, trees and pollens, before choosing this oil.

Primary use: It works as a terrific antiseptic and antifungal solution. Nails: This is great for any nail care needs when dealing with fungus. Skin: Perfect for treating dry, cracked hands or feet. It also works on dry, mature, wrinkled conditions. Hair: It is added to solutions to make brittle hair have more moisture.

SPEARMINT   (top note) Its minty aroma makes it a hit with most people. It has an uplifting effect to clients just walking in. Some salons choose to use this oil as a natural fragrance to brighten up the atmosphere.

Primary use: Besides using its natural aroma to uplift the room, it is used as a body toning oil.

TAGETES   (base note) **CAUTION:** This essential oil must be used with extreme care. It is toxic if used directly on the skin, hands and feet. Never use during pregnancy, as it has a naturally abortive reaction.)

Primary use: With all the warnings of its being toxic, if used in a very diluted blend, it is extremely effective when treating athlete's foot and any fungal infections of the nails.

TEA TREE   (top note) This essential oil has a very pungent aroma, and, by itself, is not particularly appealing. It has strong antiseptic and antifungal properties, and works well in all areas of the body.

Primary use: Hair: On the scalp it is very effective in controlling dandruff and any irritations. Skin: Improves acne conditions and reduces excess sebum. It is one of nature's best ointments for herpes. Nails: It works incredibly well to control nail fungus.

THYME (Sweet and Lemon)   (top note) Both oils work very well as antibiotics, antiseptics, and antifungals.

Primary use: Due to their special properties, they are extremely effective during a pedicure. Treats any fungal infections on the nails, hands and feet. Used as an antiseptic for the scalp and skin.

VIOLET LEAF   (middle note) It has a very light and pleasant aroma, which makes it particularly favorable with mature women. It is a relatively mild oil.

Primary use: Skin and nails: It is used to moisturize skin on the body, face, hands, and feet. It softens the appearance of wrinkles on mature skin.

YLANG-YLANG   (base note) The grades of oil available for aromatherapy are of a lesser quality. They tend to resemble jasmine in fragrance, although not quite as distinct. Its aroma can be repelling to some; therefore, check with your client before adding it to the blend. As in all tree oils, check for allergies to tree pollens before deciding to use this essential oil.

Primary use: Hair: It helps to degrease oily hair and scalp. Skin: Can help control acne and oily skin conditions. Nails: During pedicures, ylang-ylang acts to soften rough calluses.

Appendix C

Quick Reference to the 17 Base (Carrier) Oils

1. Almond Oil
2. Apricot Kernel Oil
3. Avocado Oil
4. Borage Seed Oil
5. Hazelnut Oil
6. Carrot Oil
7. Corn Oil
8. Evening Primrose Oil
9. Grapeseed Oil
10. Jojoba Oil
11. Olive Oil
12. Peanut Oil
13. Safflower Oil
14. Sesame Oil
15. Soya Bean Oil
16. Sunflower Oil
17. Wheatgerm Oil

Appendix D

Notes and References

Preface

1. "Crisis healing," a term used during a personal conversation between Mario Montalvo and Shelley M. Hess (author) on January 29, 1995. Montalvo used this expression to describe the prevalent reaction to essential oils during the very first treatment. **NOTE:** This is not a copyrighted/trademarked term.

2. During a lecture on "Homopathic Skin Analysis" at the Long Beach Guild's trade show (January 28–30, 1995), Mario Montalvo demonstrated to the audience this easy way to test if the client will have a greater chance to have a "crisis healing" experience. For the purpose of this book, I am calling it the "toxicity test." **NOTE:** This is not a copyrighted/trademarked term.

Chapter 2

1. Montalvo, Mario. "Origins in Use of Botanical Ingredients." *Dermascope* (Nov.–Dec. 1994): 70.

Chapter 3

1. In addition to using my own personal experiences working with the essential oils to determine oil categories, the following two sources were also used:

   Lavabre, Marcel. *Aromatherapy Workbook*. Rochester, VT: Healing Arts Press, 1990.

   Price, Shirley. *Practical Aromatherapy*. London: Thorsons Publishing, 1983.

Chapter 7

1. Worwood, Valerie A. *The Complete Book of Essential Oils on Aromatherapy*. San Rafael, CA: New World Library, 1995.

Chapter 8

1. "Clinical Trials on the Influence of Cigarette Fumes on Dermatological Conditions." *Society of Cosmetic Chemists Journal* (June 1991).

2. Wildwood, Christine. "Holistic Aromatherapy." *Les Nouvelles Esthetiques* (Dec. 1994): 40.

Index

Notes

Notes

Style.
Savvy.
Solutions.

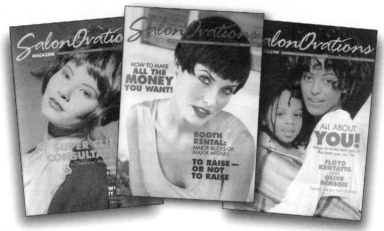

every month.
SalonOvations

SalonOvations is a professional and personal magazine designed with you in mind. Each issue delivers great features on personal growth and on-target stories about the beauty business. Get helpful hints from industry pros on starting your own salon business and how to satisfy your clients. Plus, you'll get pages of colorful photos of the latest trends in haircutting, styling and coloring.

All this at a great price of 12 **15** issues for only $19.95 a year! **3 FREE issues** - Save over 40%

(price subject to change)